PSYCHIATRIC INTERVIEWING

A Primer

Second Edition

D1235697

PSYCHIATRIC INTERVIEWING

A Primer

Second Edition

Robert L. Leon, MD

Professor and Chairman
Department of Psychiatry
The University of Texas Health Science Center at San Antonio

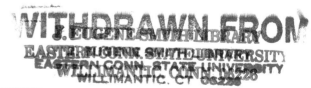

Elsevier
New York • Amsterdam • London

Elsevier Science Publishing Co., Inc.
655 Avenue of the Americas, New York, New York 10010

Sole distributors outside the United States and Canada:
Elsevier Science Publishers B.V.
P.O. Box 211, 1000 AE Amsterdam, the Netherlands

© 1989 by Elsevier Science Publishing Co., Inc.

This book has been registered with the Copyright Clearance Center, Inc.
For further information, please contact the Copyright Clearance Center, Inc.,
Salem, Massachusetts.

Library of Congress Cataloging-in-Publication Data

Leon, Robert L.
    Psychiatric interviewing : a primer / Robert L. Leon.—2nd ed.
        p.   cm.
    Includes bibliographies and index.
    ISBN 0-444-01332-6
    1. Interviewing in psychiatry. I. Title.
    [DNLM: 1. Interview, Psychological—methods. 2. Physician–Patient
Relations. WM 141 L579p]
    RC480.7.L46 1989
    616.89'0751—dc19
DNLM/DLC
for Library of Congress   88-21271
                                      CIP

Current printing (last digit)
10 9 8 7 6 5 4 3 2 1

Manufactured in the United States of America

Dedicated to the discipline
of an open mind

Contents

Preface

The original purpose of the first edition of this book was to outline the process of psychiatric interviewing and to give the reader some vicarious experience with interviewing patients by using selected examples. The book deals with questions that come to mind as patients are interviewed and gives a "road map" to follow for the examination. It has proved useful in helping medical students learn to interview patients, primarily those on the psychiatric service. In addition, reviewers and those using the book have commented on its value to residents in psychiatry and family practice and to physicians in general. Since the first edition went to press, there has been more emphasis in the medical literature on the importance of physicians listening to and understanding their patients.

Physicians are confronted with research studies that show that doctors do not listen to their patients and do not respond to much of what patients say to them. These studies also show that patients want more than technical competence from their doctors. They want communication, understanding, and empathy. They also want to understand and participate in their medical care.

This second edition, while retaining the format and material of the first edition, has been expanded to incorporate some new material on how physicians relate to patients, new research on interviewing, and material describing a more structured approach to interviewing that is now being used to complement the basic approach described in the book. Other material has been added that should make the book more useful to the practicing physician and the resident-in-training while still maintaining value for the medical student.

Again, I want to thank those who contributed the sections of the book that bear their names. Thanks also to Martin B. Giffen, MD, and to Ms. Diana Schiller. A number of residents and faculty of the Department of Psychiatry reviewed all or parts of the book and made helpful comments.

Contributors

David S. Fuller, MD
Professor and Chief
Liaison-Consultation Service
Department of Psychiatry
The University of Texas Health Science Center at San
    Antonio
San Antonio, Texas

Robert L. Leon, MD
Professor and Chairman
Department of Psychiatry
The University of Texas Health Science Center at San
    Antonio
San Antonio, Texas

Cervando Martinez, Jr, MD
Professor
Department of Psychiatry
The University of Texas Health Science Center at San
    Antonio
San Antonio, Texas

James M. Turnbull, MD, FRCP(C)
Professor and Chairman
Department of Psychiatry and Behavioral Sciences
Quillen-Dishner College of Medicine
East Tennessee State University
Johnson City, Tennessee

1

Introduction

This is a book about interviewing and the therapeutic doctor–patient relationship as it applies to medical practice. It is a book about how the doctor can get to know patients as unique individuals and use the doctor–patient relationship as an important tool for both evaluation and therapy. It is written for doctors and those studying to become doctors, but the basic principles can be applied by all health care professionals in their work with patients.

The book is a culmination of many years of working with medical students, residents in psychiatry, and other doctors to help them learn to interview patients on psychiatric, medical, and surgical services who have serious problems that they want to discuss with their doctors. They may be patients in deep depression, or those who have severe and intolerable anxiety that may make no sense to them, but is there, nevertheless. They may be patients with an organic disease that they do not understand and are therefore desperately afraid of what may be happening to their bodies. They may be patients who complain of physical symptoms, but whose real problems stem from emotional stress caused by an unbearable living situation.

Whoever they are, they all need one of the most important persons in their lives at that moment—their doctor—to listen, understand, and give support. The patient's talking and the doctor's listening still remain one of the most important tools for making a diagnosis and beginning a therapeutic regimen.

During this century the advances in scientific medicine have been spectacular. In the last decade the rate of new discovery in biochemistry, molecular biology, and physiology has been escalating, but much of the new science does not lead to a better understanding of the patient as a person and his or her feelings of distress. It remains for the doctor to achieve this understanding through the skilled use of the doctor–

patient relationship. The doctor has the responsibility to develop this relationship and use it in guiding the patient through the diagnostic and therapeutic process.

Since the responsibility for creating and maintaining the doctor–patient relationship falls most heavily on the doctor, he or she must have some guidance in how to develop this relationship in a manner that will both enlist patient participation and permit the doctor to obtain the necessary information for diagnosis and treatment.

The patient's welfare is the first concern and the major reason for improving interviewing skills. But there is another reason: the doctor's satisfaction and pride in doing a job well. An expertly and sensitively developed doctor–patient relationship allows the doctor to understand his or her patients in a way that will surely enhance satisfaction in the practice of medicine, emotional and intellectual satisfaction in being a better diagnostician and therapist, and emotional satisfaction in having developed a professionally controlled relationship with patients. Dealing with the emotional and intellectual aspects of doctor, patient, and the doctor–patient relationship is built into the plan of this book.

It is written from a psychiatric perspective. This perspective allows us to understand the patient in that person's social, psychological, and physical being. The art and science of interviewing has been more highly developed by psychiatry than any other medical specialty. Nevertheless, many examples were taken from other fields of medicine to demonstrate how this approach is useful to all doctors, no matter what their specialty.

In the second chapter, I discuss the doctor–patient relationship. There is much anecdotal and scientific evidence of the power of this relationship.

Freud understood this and attempted to control the relationship so that the patient's inner conflicts could emerge (Freud 1966). Balint studied the relationship as it applied to general medical practice (Balint 1957). Cousins stated it in this way: ". . . the physician is not just a prescriber of medicaments but a symbol of all transferable from one human to another, short of immortality" (Cousins 1981). With an awareness of the power and limitations of the relationship and some knowledge of how it develops, one is ready to meet the patient.

The next chapter deals with the specifics of meeting the patient and starting the interview. How the interviewer introduces himself or herself and addresses the patient may seem to be small things, but they set the tone of the relationship. The doctor's opening remarks are crucial. The patient hangs on every word and carefully follows the doctor's perceived instructions. I will discuss what to say and what to look for at this important early stage.

After the interview is underway, the clinician must keep it going so that patients can say what is on their minds and so the doctor can obtain necessary information. This is a formidable task. The chapter on the body of the interview gives examples of how to accomplish this. In this chapter I discuss important verbal and nonverbal information to be obtained, as well as present a more formal discussion of psychiatric history and mental status examination. This discussion of psychiatric history and mental status examination is one of the parts of the book most related to psychiatry. Even so, doctors in many specialties are called on to make a psychiatric evaluation from time to time, either because no psychiatrist is available or in order to aid in making a psychiatric referral. This section should be of interest to all reading the book, and it certainly will be helpful to medical students during their rotation on psychiatry.

After the opening and a period of exploration, most interviews must be ended in some way. The chapter on closing includes ways to do this and covers a problem unique to medical students and housestaff: what to say to patients when the student leaves the service.

In several chapters I review some special situations that require a modification of the basic approach to interviewing discussed earlier in the book. Some patients, such as those with great anxiety or those with concrete thinking, must be approached differently. I also discuss how to respond to special problems such as a patient's crying or asking for advice.

Through the years, I have observed that students, and even experienced interviewers, make certain predictable mistakes as they open and conduct an interview. These are reviewed in the chapter on some common pitfalls.

Interviewing family members and the family as a group has become an important part of psychiatric evaluation and therapy. This requires a somewhat different technique and approach. One needs to obtain the patient's permission to talk with the family or family members, and then one must carefully consider what to tell the family about the patient's illness. When conducting family interviews, physicians have a different level of activity and make different observations than when conducting individual interviews.

Every encounter a physician has with a patient has potential therapeutic value. Some knowledge of the basic elements of psychotherapy will give the clinician a better understanding of the therapeutic elements in each interview. The examples at the end of the section on psychotherapy show its potential value. This chapter will give all physicians a deeper understanding of how the so-called ''talking therapies'' work. It also gives a few rudimentary principles and some caveats that will aid those who want to extend therapeutic interviewing beyond the evaluation phase.

The chapter, "An Organizing Framework," has been added to help in ordering and integrating the vast amount of information that can be obtained from and about a person.

Little technical language is used in this book because I believe the use of technical language detracts from one of the major purposes of the book—to give the reader some flavor of the interview and of the doctor–patient relationship. Numerous excerpts from actual interviews and the epilogue have been included to help the reader experience the interview process. Many good textbooks of psychiatry and other more specialized books adequately present technical material.

Working with patients is a fascinating experience. It is one reason why most people go into medicine. Unfortunately, much of medical education does not impart the knowledge, techniques, trials and tribulations, and joys of this experience. This book is an attempt to do so.

References

Balint M: *The Doctor, His Patient and the Illness*. New York, International Universities Press, 1957.

Cousins N: The physician in literature. *Saturday Review*, February 1981, p 8.

Freud S: *The Standard Edition of the Complete Psychological Works of Sigmund Freud. The Dynamics of Transference*, vol 12. London, Hogarth Press, 1966.

2

The Doctor–Patient Relationship

Art, Science, and Therapy in the Interview

Interviewing is an art, a science, and a therapeutic tool all wrapped up in one complex package. It is not a diffuse activity to be carried out willy-nilly with little thought, but rather to obtain specific information. It has a beginning, a middle, and an end. The interviewer who understands the structure will find, as have artists in other fields, that medical interviewing can be a satisfying mode of self-expression if the finished product has a clarity that can be appreciated by others.

Although this book is designed to help the student learn interviewing, from time to time I will stress that knowledge of the psychodynamics of interpersonal relationships and personality is the basic science for treating all patients as people with illnesses. By learning the basic principles of the interview, students and physicians will learn to relate better to all medical patients and to understand mental processes that influence illness. Information gathered through interviewing provides a primary data base for a total medical psychodynamic diagnosis.

A psychological evaluation by the physician should be a part of every comprehensive medical evaluation. Does the patient have incapacitating emotional problems? Is anxiety a problem that needs therapy and, if so, what kind? Most primary-care physicians treat psychiatric problems. These are usually mild-to-moderate anxieties and depressions, and they are often treated by medication. Before a prescription is given, a brief psychiatric evaluation should be made and the physician should consider the therapeutic aspects of the doctor–patient relationship in planning treatment. Used properly, this may prove superior to medication.

Unfortunately, many otherwise knowledgeable physicians have never learned to develop a therapeutic relationship with their patients:

a relationship that will help relieve a patient's anxiety and fear and, at the same time, aid the physician in diagnosis and treatment. With a therapeutic doctor–patient relationship a patient can better provide the physician with necessary history and information about symptoms and is better able and more willing to participate in treatment.

In these times there are several factors that tend to overpower the human side of medicine and work against developing a therapeutic doctor–patient relationship. Medicine is becoming more commercialized; doctors are often referred to as providers, and patients as consumers or clients. At the same time, advances in science and technology are assuming greater and greater importance on medical practice. To highlight the importance of the patient in this changing medical world, medical educators have begun to put more emphasis on the interpersonal and human side of medicine where values, attitudes, and interviewing skills are basic.

Lipkin and colleagues present a core curriculum for teaching medical interviewing to residents in internal medicine. They state, "A fundamental characteristic of internal medicine is the intelligent, sensitive, and systematic collection of information from patients in various settings. The medical interview is one of the most important tools in this process. We define the interview as the entire medium of patient–physician interaction. During the interview the internist undertakes several tasks simultaneously. The internist approaches the patient as a unique person with his own story to tell, promotes trust and confidence, clarifies and characterizes the patient's symptoms and concerns, generates and tests many hypotheses that may include biological and psychosocial dimensions of illness, and creates the basis for an ongoing relationship."

The Power of the Doctor–Patient Relationship

All medical treatment is both physiological and psychological, and it begins with the first encounter of doctor and patient. Just making an appointment with the doctor makes some patients feel better. The feelings patients have during the course of therapy are important for recovery. For certain psychophysiological problems, working with these feelings may be the most important part of therapy.

Studies show that patients with ulcerative colitis, peptic ulcer, asthma, and other so-called psychosomatic disorders have a higher recovery rate and stay well longer when they receive a combination of pharmacological and psychotherapy than when they receive either therapy alone (Luborsky et al 1975). There may be a compound effect of drugs and psychotherapy that exceeds the simple additive effects of either.

Jensen states, "Certainly, a patient's psychophysiologic responses to the physician are no less real than responses to the drugs or other treatment prescribed by the physician (Jensen 1981). Much of the aid a physician gives a patient appears to depend upon his or her ability to mobilize the patient's positive expectations and faith within an emotionally supportive relationship."

Other studies document that a good doctor–patient relationship can determine whether a patient makes satisfactory or unsatisfactory progress (Rosenstock 1975). The doctor–patient relationship is an important factor in the patient's reaction to postoperative pain (Egbert et al 1964). In the treatment of chronic diseases such as diabetes, doctor and patient must cooperate fully to manage the illness. Before scientific medicine, the main tool doctors had was their presence at the bedside.

Sometimes an adequate explanation within the context of a trusting doctor–patient relationship can take the place of medication. A woman who had been receiving psychoactive medication for several years as a regular patient in a psychiatric clinic came in stating that she was pregnant. The doctor assigned to her for regular prescription refills in a busy medication clinic recommended that she not take the medication during her pregnancy. She refused. In order to more adequately deal with the situation, the patient was assigned to another physician who could spend more time with the patient. After two interviews, during which a relationship was formed and the patient was allowed to express her fears of what would happen if she stopped her medication, she agreed to stop after a phased reduction. She continues to do well while seeing her doctor regularly.

Michael Balint stated this principle: ". . . by far the most frequently used drug in general practice was the doctor himself, i.e., that it was not only the bottle of medicine or the box of pills that mattered, but the way the doctor gave them to his patient—in fact the whole atmosphere in which the drug was given and taken" (Balint 1957).

The belief system of the doctor and patient is so important that research into the efficacy of new drugs cannot be accepted unless the study is carried out "double blind"—that is, some patients receive a placebo or another medication and other patients receive the drug to be tested. The drugs are made up and dispensed in such a way that neither the doctor nor the patient knows which is the active ingredient. Some designs are even more sophisticated and incorporate the double-blind cross-over technique. At some predetermined time the active and inactive medications are switched without the knowledge of either the patient or the attending physician. Doctors and the Food and Drug Administration have all learned not to accept the supposed therapeutic benefits of any new drug that has not been tested by methods designed to minimize the powerful influences of the doctor–patient interaction.

Since double-blind therapeutic drug trials are so important, we are forced to conclude that the physician's feelings influence not only the patient's therapeutic response to the drug but also the physician's perception of that response. Doctors' perceptions are often colored by the feelings aroused in them by the patient. These feelings, if used constructively and with insight, can be a diagnostic and therapeutic tool rather than an obstacle to good, objective patient care.

The Doctor's Reactions

Within the relationship of the interview, feelings inevitably develop within the doctor. These are often ignored or dismissed as inappropriate. Even worse, the doctor may feel guilty about these feelings. Yet feelings may serve as an important diagnostic tool. Depressed people arouse feelings of depression in others even if the depressed person is trying to smile. Rumke has gone so far as to say that the only valid diagnostic criterion for schizophrenia is the "precox feeling." This is an intuitive experience that the examiner has that it is impossible to empathize with the patient. He stated that only those patients with whom one cannot establish an empathic relationship should be diagnosed as schizophrenic (Rumke 1957). Although the diagnosis of schizophrenia or any other disease should not be dependent on the doctor's feelings, Rumke's "precox feeling" is an example of the importance of these feelings.

Smith did a study of medical students' interviewing techniques that demonstrated that the students' feelings do make a difference in the material covered in the interview. Students who had been previously noted to have adequate interview skills were observed during interviews in which they were instructed to obtain "the history of the present illness in its psychosocial as well as biological dimensions in 30 minutes" (Smith 1984). During the sessions, the author watched for countertransference behavior, which was defined as behavior that was potentially harmful to the interview (e.g., avoiding significant topics or showing disrespect). In the postinterview discussion it was possible to link these potentially harmful behaviors to feelings the students had that were not based on reality (such as avoiding certain topics because the student feared harming the patient, or because he or she feared losing control). The student was often unaware of these feelings until the discussion following the interview.

Of the 15 students whose interviews were carefully reviewed, 13 showed countertransference behavior and 14 demonstrated countertransference feelings during the postinterview discussion. In no instance was the student fully aware of the underlying behavior and feelings. The most common behavior was avoiding psychosocial issues.

Students also avoided areas related to physical symptoms because of their own fears. One student avoided all questions involving gastrointestinal symptoms in a jaundiced patient of the student's same age because the student felt the patient might have cancer and did not want to find out, and because of the student's own fear that a growth the student had might be cancer. This demonstrates that students' feelings are real and do influence the interview.

Feelings can give clues to diagnosis or important characteristics in other patients. Manic patients, when they are not hostile, can be amusing and produce good feelings in their doctor. A feeling of rejection aroused in the doctor may signal one of the patient's problems—stimulating rejection in others. Manifestations of the doctor's feelings have even been described as an objective sign. Ascher's sign is the clenching of the doctor's fist while he or she is listening to the history given by an hysteric patient. Although the validity of Ascher's sign should be questioned, the importance of understanding the doctor's response to patients is beyond question.

The doctor who ignores his or her own feelings is rejecting an important diagnostic tool: experiencing directly the reaction that the patient stimulates in others. These feelings may be just as significant as anything observed in a physical examination of a patient. A patient may come to the doctor complaining of shortness of breath. If, during the physical examination, a heart murmur, enlarged heart, or edema of the legs are found, one concludes that the patient has a cardiac problem. If expiratory wheezes are heard in the lungs, asthma is suspected. Using one's own feelings to help diagnose depression or schizophrenia is more subtle and not nearly so reliable as the findings during physical examination, but these feelings should nevertheless be treated as data to be used with other information in the total assessment of the patient. More sophisticated and knowledgeable physicians can use feelings to learn more about how patients may relate to others.

Physicians should also try to be more aware of their own feelings in order to gain more insight into their own personality and prejudices. Earlier we cited studies that show that medical students may have feelings that greatly interfered with their ability to conduct a satisfactory interview. Anxiety over performance or unpleasant emotions aroused by unpleasant subjects would cause the student to abruptly change topics or completely avoid further questioning in these unpleasant areas (Smith 1984). Physicians have the responsibility to be aware of these and other emotions in themselves. They should, as much as possible, be alert to stimuli from patients that cause unreasonably angry, nurturing, or amorous feelings. We do not say physicians must rid themselves of all emotional responses. That would be impossible;

however, they should be alert to feelings so that they will not interfere with the doctor–patient relationship.

Some Dilemmas in the Doctor–Patient Interaction

An interview has two important functions: One is to create an atmosphere for mutual exploration in which the patient feels free to say what is on his or her mind; the second is to obtain information necessary for diagnosis and treatment. Creating an atmosphere for relaxed discussion while maintaining an orderly progression toward a complete history and mental status examination poses an early dilemma for students. This problem exists in every evaluation, and particularly in a psychiatric evaluation—even for the sophisticated. An interview is not a casual conversation and should not be treated as such by either the doctor or patient. Nevertheless, a relaxed atmosphere is to be encouraged.

Usually, the patient expects to be asked questions and, indeed, the doctor has many questions in mind. Herein lies another problem: how to get necessary information without asking too many questions and thus stopping the conversation. Specific questions will elicit specific information, but they also tend to halt free-flowing conversation or get the patient off the track. Most of us have had the experience of joining a group at a party and asking a question tangential to the topic of conversation. The question is answered, but the conversation then stops while the group tried to get back on the original track.

On first contact with a physician, a patient waits for clues from the doctor that tell him or her how to respond. The doctor gives these clues both verbally and nonverbally. Nonverbal clues are given by facial expression and body position. For example, the interviewer can show greater interest by leaning forward. If the doctor relaxes and looks out of the window, the patient may take this to mean that the doctor is not interested. Doctors, as well as patients, give clues of which they are unaware. Here are two examples, taken from videotaped interviews, of verbal clues given by the doctor. The interviews will be presented in more detail later. Even though I will mostly by discussing verbal clues, keep in mind that nonverbal clues given by the doctor may be even more powerful in determining a patient's behavior in an interview:

> DOCTOR: You might start by telling me *how you got into the hospital*.
>
> PATIENT: How I got into the hospital . . .

Another patient:

> DOCTOR: . . . what has been happening to you *lately* . . . why don't you just *start* out . . .
>
> PATIENT: *Start lately?* Well, *lately* . . .

The striking thing about the responses of both patients is that the patients began their history by using almost the exact words of the doctor's opening statement: "How I got into the hospital . . ." and "Start lately?" The doctor's opening remarks are a potent factor in determining the direction and content of the interview. Interviewers might keep this in mind and analyze the patient's opening remarks as a response to their opening statement or question. In the examples above, the doctor's opening statement could have been a more specific question rather than a general invitation to the patient to start talking.

Even in this early stage of the interview, the two aforementioned functions of the interview (encouraging the patient to say whatever is on his or her mind, and obtaining necessary information) are already in conflict. These functions are not incompatible: They just seem so at times, especially when there is a limited amount of time, several patients to see, and information to be recorded on the chart. Students should be reassured that research demonstrates that patients, if allowed to talk, do present most necessary information. Cox and colleagues found that mothers who brought their children for psychiatric evaluation mentioned almost all important problems when encouraged to talk spontaneously (Cox et al 1981).

If we keep in mind that some of the most important facts are the problems of interpersonal relationships as perceived by the patient, this dilemma all but disappears. We need to hear the patient's view of the world as uncontaminated as possible by questions, prodding, and cajoling from the physician. Adolt Meyer, one of the founding fathers of modern American psychiatry, is supposed to have said, "Facts are anything which make a difference" (Meyer 1948). If a patient believes that his wife is being unfaithful to him, it will make a big difference in how he feels about her whether or not she actually is unfaithful. It may even cause the patient to come to the physician with some seemingly unrelated physical problem because he cannot express his real feelings openly.

Frequently we see more subtle misperceptions that determine behavior that provokes responses in others that seem to "prove" the misperception. For example, a person expects a phone call from a friend, but the friend was unexpectedly busy with something else. The next time the two friends meet, the first person may be somewhat hostile and thus provoke a withdrawal on the part of the friend. This confirms the first person's belief that the friend did not want to make the expected call. If a patient discusses such a situation in an interview, you might be tempted to dismiss it with a statement such as, "Maybe you were wrong about why your friend didn't call." If so, you would have missed the essential point, which would be the person's feelings about himself or herself as not being likeable. Similarly, in the first example, the man may feel inadequate and that is why he believes his wife is being unfaithful to him.

What patients think is happening will determine their behavior, and what they think may be determined more by their feelings about themselves than by external reality. These feelings represent an internal reality to be explored. This internal psychological reality is the cornerstone of psychiatric data.

> Data gathering from humans has been hampered by the fact that a great deal of evaluative function occurs in the brain without awareness. Indeed important emotional conflicts are likely to be shunted out of awareness. . . . The information remains in the brain, however, perfectly capable of being recruited on appropriate stimulation and entering the complex process of behavior. (Wolf and Goodell 1979)

These are difficult concepts for those oriented to the world of experimental science, numbers, and "external reality." Just remember that many of the "facts" are in the mind of the patient, and the doctor's job is to create an atmosphere in which these can be expressed freely with no fear of criticism.

In successful psychotherapy, patients' internal perceptions begin to approximate external reality. One patient, after a long period of psychotherapy, was reviewing the progress she had made. She said, "I'm not bitter now, but I used to be bitter toward everybody. I didn't like anyone. It seemed as if what happened to me was always someone else's fault. In my confusion I couldn't see that it was my fault, that my family was not inviting me over on holidays because I was so hostile. Now I can reason things out. I can see things more clearly." It took a long time for this woman to work through her conflicts and begin to understand that her hostility stemmed from her feelings of abandonment by her mother, who died when the patient was four years old. If her doctor had questioned her perceptions early in therapy, she would never have felt free to explore and later express her deeper feelings about the death of her mother.

The thoughts and feelings of the patient are the "facts" that will make up much of the psychiatric data to be recorded in the chart and used to formulate diagnosis and treatment. These thoughts and feelings must come from the patient's mind and not from preconceived notions of the interviewer. Doctors cannot be certain about what is on a patient's mind until a patient chooses to tell them. In some cases, patients themselves are not entirely aware of what is troubling them. During the course of an interview, thoughts, feelings, and statements may come forth that surprise a patient. Slips of the tongue sometimes reveal thoughts and feelings hitherto unknown to a patient. Patients may be aware of other things that they are reluctant to discuss, and they look for an excuse not to discuss them. If the doctor is always asking questions, the patient is further relieved of the responsibility of introducing these difficult topics.

If the atmosphere of the interview is one of mutual exploration, the physician is privileged to share the patient's thoughts and feelings. In our society the opportunities for this sharing are rare, but if patients feel accepted, they share their thoughts and feelings—at least to the best of their ability—with their physician. There is probably no other situation in which this occurs.

The Open Mind

The first component in helping to open a patient's mind to the doctor, and at the same time to the patient himself, is the interviewer's mind set. The doctor must enter the situation accepting what the patient brings, and from there help the patient bring out what he or she considers to be important. Patients are willing—at times eager—to tell about themselves and their problems, but they must first feel that this material will be well received by the listener. The interviewer does not have to agree with the patient, support his or her viewpoints, or condone the patient's previous actions. The physician must, however, listen nonjudgmentally and convey to the patient that he or she is eager to understand how the patient sees the world. Patients do not usually expect their doctor to agree with them, but they do expect that they will hear them out and not judge them adversely. When judgment is passed, the patient becomes defensive and the opportunity to learn of another person and their perception of the world may be lost.

To remain open, the interviewer must always be aware of preconceived ideas. For example, a medical student interviewing a 22-year-old woman asked about her children and learned that she had two sons, aged two and five years. Later in the interview the woman said she had been married for three years. At this point the student became embarrassed and changed the subject. The student's beliefs about out-of-wedlock pregnancies caused the embarrassment. The woman may not have been concerned about the time discrepancies. She may have been married twice or she may not consider having a child out of wedlock to be a problem, but we never learned. The interviewer's attitudes and feelings indirectly stopped communication.

Freeling and Harris found that assumptions influence the doctor–patient relationship (Freeling and Harris 1984). If the assumptions of the doctor do not closely approximate those of the patient, the relationship is unduly complicated. It, therefore, behooves the doctor to learn as much as possible about the patient's assumptions about what medical consultation may offer to the patient. The doctor cannot always assume what a patient wants or what upsets a patient. This is illustrated in an example given by Freeling and Harris from an English practitioner's consultations:

> Wendy Acheson, aged 22, came into the consulting room, and before she had even reached the chair, said to the doctor, "The bastard! He's done it again!"
>
> It appeared that her husband had just told her that he had been found to have gonorrhoea, and wanted her to get some treatment. It was the third time that this happened, and on each occasion the infection had followed one of his business trips to Birmingham.
>
> "What are you going to do?" asked the doctor. "I suppose I'd better have some more Septrin." Thinking of the problems that even one such announcement might have caused in some marriages, the doctor was a little surprised at her reaction. (Freeling and Harris 1984, p 18)

One might assume that Mrs. Acheson would want to explore the relationship with her husband, and well she might, but not necessarily so. She may accept things as they are. It would be unwise for the doctor to burden her with his or her own assumptions or proceed to act on them without first reconciling them with those of the patient.

To be nonjudgmental, to be aware of one's feelings, to be able to say nothing or the right thing at the right time is asking a lot of any student or a physician. All of this may at first seem impossible, but as with any skill or talent, knowledge and practice produce good performance. Some people, more than others, have a greater native ability to develop interpersonal skills, one of which is interviewing. Some are especially talented at recognizing the nuances of nonverbal communication and also may give constructive nonverbal, but unconscious, feedback. Others may have a background that demands close attention to and anticipation of another's reaction. Most of us can develop therapeutic doctor–patient relationships, but the ability is latent and must be cultivated. Interviewing is a skill one develops throughout one's lifetime. Each time a doctor sees a patient, he or she will learn a little more about that patient, more about doctor–patient relations, and more about himself or herself. A doctor's first obligation is to the patient, but try to remember that, with each encounter, an added benefit is learning more about oneself.

The Setting

We use the term "setting" to include the whole ambience of the interview, not just the physical setting although that is also important.

The importance of the setting cannot be overestimated. For example, society and culture can influence people for better or worse. It has been demonstrated that societal changes can produce an increased incidence of hypertension and other cardiovascular diseases. In their study of Roseto, Pennsylvania, a study that spanned more than 15 years, Bruhn and Wolf concluded that susceptibility to myocardial infarction and sudden death increased as the support system from family and friends decreased (Bruhn and Wolf 1979). From 1887, when Roseto was founded, until the 1960s, the people of that community had maintained a close-knit social life centered around family, church, and community. At times of crisis, family and friends had given emotional and material support. Although there had been differences in wealth, those who had money had not displayed it through extravagant living. During this period, death by myocardial infarction had been remarkably low— approaching that of rural Italy from which the town's people came. In the 1960s, the citizens of Roseto began relating more to nearby communities and taking on the values of the larger world. Family and community ties loosened and support systems decreased. Myocardial infarction rates began to approach those of other communities.

There are other examples of the importance of the social, cultural, and psychological environment. For example, a significantly higher incidence of all types of illness and accidents follow traumatic life events. The most traumatic are the death of a spouse or parent. Statistical studies show that major medical problems often occur in the survivors (Holmes 1978). Other studies document how patients in a mental hospital will act out—that is, behave badly or destructively— in response to unspoken feelings and conflicts of doctors and nurses (Stanton and Schwartz 1954).

In a similar way, patients will consciously and unconsciously respond to the feelings of their doctor and those around them. A busy clinic with insufficient privacy is not the best place to conduct an interview, but if the doctor is unperturbed and can attend to the patient, the interview may be better than in a private office with a domineering, preoccupied physician.

The setting is significant in the feelings it arouses in both the patient and the doctor. These depend for the most part on the unique perceptions of those involved: how each person interprets the situation individually. Psychiatric patients are prone to idiosyncratic interpretations of their perceptions of interpersonal relationships; this is one reason that they are psychiatric patients. Psychoanalysts call these idiosyncratic interpretations "transference" when they occur in the doctor–patient relationship. Feelings developed in an earlier relationship with a significant person, usually a parent, are transferred to the relationship with the doctor, and usually these feelings are not appropriate to the present relationship.

Transference inevitably occurs, but a more neutral setting will minimize it. A well-run clinic and a quiet office with chairs placed a respectable distance apart and not directly facing each other will respect some patients' need to keep emotional distance between themselves and the therapist. Such a setting will protect other patients from being overcome by hostile or amorous impulses.

Listening

Studies have shown over and over that students, residents, and sometimes practicing physicians do not listen to and do not respond to the concerns of their patients. Kent and colleagues (1981) found this problem in studying interviews by medical students. They offered the following example:

> PATIENT: I sometimes feel a little overprotected.

> STUDENT: Do you have any problems with your heart now?

Here the student was either not listening, or, for some reason, was reticent in responding to the patient's feelings. Several other comments would have permitted the patient to continue. Here are some examples:

> "Oh?"

> "Overprotected?"

> "Tell me more about how you feel."

In a review of more than 300 clinical interviews in a medical service, Platt and McMath found that physicians at all levels had many problems in their interactions with patients during interviews. A common problem is not listening to patients when they are expressing feelings or discussing a symptom that is not on the doctor's "mental list" to explore at that moment (Platt and McMath 1979).

Even if the patients are willing to share, it appears not to be easy for the physicians to accept this. Some physicians—all of us sometimes—do not want to know that much about another person. Doctors may not like what they, themselves, are feeling in response to what patients say. This is why it is so much easier to keep an interview on a "factual" basis: When did the illness begin? How long has the patient been hospitalized? But, as we have said, feelings are facts too. Feelings engendered in the doctors who empathize with patients and want to help them improve their lives are also facts and have a profound influence on treatment. Some patients have so many problems that it is difficult to see a solution: a 23-year-old woman who had her first of five children at age 14 and whose older husband (44 years of age) is disabled; a 16-year-old unmarried mother living with her parents and caring for her own 18-month-old child as well as a 3-year-old sister with cerebral palsy. So doctors cut off communication in subtle unconscious ways and may miss forever that rare opportunity to encourage patients to express what is on their minds and to use the understanding so gained in a helpful way. Sometimes all one can do is listen, but this in itself can be therapeutic.

An extreme example of how doctors' feelings may influence judgment occurs every day in medical practice with patients who have multiple physical complaints for which no definitive cause or satisfactory treatment can be found. These patients arouse feelings of guilt and anger in their physicians. Out of physicians' efforts to be more helpful, many of these patients are referred for surgery. Many have repeated surgery, each operation being an attempt to find the cause for the patient's complaints. For some of these patients, having a doctor who would listen to their complaints might have been the only therapy needed. Some patients would have at least felt better if they were allowed to talk about their symptoms.

Malan and colleagues studied patients who were seen for psychiatric evaluation but never received treatment (Malan et al 1975). Many of these patients reported improvement after one interview. Some of these patients were followed for as long as ten years. Not all patients seen for one interview improved, but, of those who did, there were some powerful therapeutic effects. The interview helped them gain a better understanding of themselves by the self-analysis that was obtained from the discussion and also brought them face-to-face with the necessity to take some responsibility for their own lives.

Patients, after having completed what their doctor considers to be a diagnostic interview, will often say, "I feel better now that I have told you this." Talking has helped, but listening is the other half of that process. Patients will not talk if their doctors do not listen, and listening is active, not passive. Therapeutic listening requires that the doctor be attuned to what the patient says, monitor his or her own feelings, and anticipate his or her own responses and how these may affect the patient.

The doctor–patient relationship remains a part of the art of medicine. It is a disciplined relationship, but within its bounds physicians can express their own personality in approaching patients. A successful interview can begin if physicians are aware of all the forces in the doctor–patient relationship including their own feelings and responses.

References

Balint M: *The Doctor, His Patient and the Illness*. New York, International Universities Press, 1957.

Bruhn JG, Wolf S: *The Roseto Story: An Anatomy of Health*. Norman, Oklahoma, University of Oklahoma Press, 1979.

Cousins N: The physician in literature. *Saturday Review,* February 1981, p 8.

Cox A, Rutter M, Holbrook D: Psychiatric interviewing techniques V. Experimental study: eliciting factual information. *Br J Psychiatry* 1981;139:29–37.

Egbert LD, Battit GE, Welch CE, Bartlett MK: Reduction of postoperative pain by encouragement and instruction of patients. *N Engl J Med* 1964;270:825–827.

Freeling P, Harris CM: *The Doctor–Patient Relationship,* 3rd ed. Edinburgh, London, Melbourne, New York, Churchill Livingstone, 1984.

Holmes T: Life situations, emotions, and disease. *Psychosomatics* 1978;19:747–754.

Jensen PS: The doctor–patient relationship: headed for impasse or improvement? *Ann Intern Med* 1981;95:769–771.

Kent GG, Clark P, Dalrymple-Smith D: The patient is the expert: a technique for teaching interviewing skills. *J Med Educ* 1981;15:38–42.

Lipkin M Jr, Quill TE, Napodano RJ: The medical interview: a core curriculum for residencies in internal medicine. *Ann Intern Med* 1984;100(2):277–284.

Luborsky L, Singer B, Luborsky L: Comparative studies of psychotherapies. *Arch Gen Psychiatry* 1975;32:995–1008.

Maguire GP, Rutter DR: History-taking for medical students I—Deficiencies in performance. *Lancet,* Sept 11, 1976, pp 556–558.

Malan DH, Heath ES, Bacal HA, Balfour FHG: Psychodynamic changes in untreated neurotic patients: II. Apparently genuine improvements. *Arch Gen Psychiatry* 1975;32:110–126.

Meyer A: *The Commonsense Psychiatry.* Lief A (ed). New York, McGraw-Hill, 1948.

Platt F, McMath JC: Clinical hypocompetence: the interview. *Ann Intern Med* 1979;91:898–902.

Rosenstock IM: Patients' compliance with health regimes. *JAMA* 1975;234:402–403.

Rumke HC: The clinical differentiation within the group of the schizophrenias, in *Proceedings of the Second International Congress of Psychiatry,* Zurich, Sept 1–7, 1957, vol 1, p 302.

Smith RC: Teaching interviewing skills to medical students: the issue of countertransference. *J Med Educ* 1984;59:582–588.

Stanton AH, Schwartz MS: *The Mental Hospital.* New York, Basic Books, 1954.

Wolf S, Goodell H: Causes and mechanisms in psychosomatic phenomena. *J Hum Stress* 1979;5:9–18.

3

Starting the Relationship

The Meeting of Doctor and Patient

The moment of encounter of doctor and patient requires the doctor's full attention. Although the physician may already have seen many patients that day, this is the first meeting of this patient and doctor. For the patient, it is important. The patient has been anticipating this meeting with a mixture of fear and hope. The patient's fear comes from many sources. What will the doctor be like? Will the patient be judged adversely? What will be found? Will the doctor want to help? The hope is that the doctor can relieve the distress. Beyond these feelings about the present situation, the first encounter with the doctor stimulates anxieties and fantasies from past relationships with parents, authority figures, and physicians.

With most patients, the balance between anxiety/fear and hope is heavily weighted on the side of hope. With some, this balance is more precarious and the first meeting can do much to tilt the feeling in one direction or another. The patient's expectation of what the doctor can do is a powerful therapeutic factor. The physician's sincere and respectful interest during this first encounter will do much to enhance this therapeutic tool. It should therefore be dealt with as an important, dignified occasion.

To begin, address the patient by name, introduce yourself, and state the purpose of the meeting. Except for special situations, use the patient's surname: This is a sign of respect. It immediately puts the patient on a more equal footing with the physician and sets the stage for mutual exploration. The patient does not call the physician by his or her first name; therefore, the interviewer should not say, "Hi, Mary" or "Hello, Sid." The interviewer says, "Hello" or "Good morning, Mrs. (or Ms.) Jones," "Hello, Mr. Smith." At what age between 13 years and 21 years one says "Come into the office, John" or "Come into the office, Mr. Doe" is open for discussion. If there is any question, it is better to err on the side of formality. Some patients may prefer to be called by their first name. This is all right if it is at their request or if it occurs later when you come to know the patient better.

Use of names is often an important indicator of social class differences; those in authority or higher position are referred to by title or surname, whereas those in lower socioeconomic situations are often called by first names. This was much more prevalent in America before recent advances toward ethnic, racial, and sexual equality. Yet, the tendency still remains to use names differently among groups and social class. Early in their education clinicians should become familiar with this tendency within themselves so that they may correct it. Every patient is entitled to the dignity of being addressed by his or her surname.

Putting the Patient at Ease

It is important to put the patient or interviewee at ease. This can sometimes be done by a casual remark as the patient is brought into the room. A comment on the weather is a good standby if nothing else comes to mind. A better comment is one more meaningful to the patient, one that acknowledges something special about them or their circumstances. An example would be, "It must be hard getting here in all this rain"—a general statement, but one that acknowledges a contribution the interviewee is making to this encounter. Others might be, "Sorry you had to wait so long," or "Was it hard to park?" Such comments can be made as the patient enters the examining room or as the doctor is closing the door. It helps to say something, but whatever is said should carry a tone appropriate to the occasion. Do not make any comments about the patient's reason for coming or about the patient's illness until you are in the privacy of the examining room.

If often helps to state the purpose of the interview, although this is not always necessary. In the emergency room patients usually know why they are there and expect a doctor to talk with them. The same is usually true in an outpatient clinic. However, a patient is sometimes brought by another person and is thus even more frightened about what will happen. This is especially true of adolescents whose parents bring them in. With these patients, a statement such as "We are just going to talk together today" is helpful. Don't start with "I'm just going to ask you some questions." I will discuss questions in more detail later.

A caveat about putting the patient at ease: When they first work with patients, medical students may overdo comments designed to put patients at ease. What the students are actually trying to do is put themselves at ease: They are more anxious than the patients. Comments such as "Sure nice of you to come," "We won't take too long," and "I hope you don't mind talking with me for a while," are not bad in themselves, but should not be used apologetically. Patients should, of course, be told that they are working with a medical student, but this can be done with some assurance that the student can be helpful.

Patients do, indeed, find interviews with medical students to be helpful even if they know that these interviews are for student training. Ries and colleagues assessed the impact of training interviews on both psychiatric patients and on the medical students who performed them. Some, but not all, of the patients found the interviews to be "very helpful." More patients than medical students felt that the interviews were worthwhile. The students found the interviews to be more stressful than the patients did, and the patients put a higher value on the interview than did the students.

Opening a Nondirective Interview

There are two kinds of interviews: directive and nondirective. These categories refer to the interviewer's communications to the patient about how the interview will progress and whether doctor or patient will determine what information will come from the interview. The terms "directive" and "nondirective" do not refer to the interview's purpose. Nondirective means allowing patients to open the interview, develop it, and proceed at their own pace. The doctor must let go yet still maintain control, which may sound paradoxical. For physicians who are overly compulsive and anxious about always doing the right thing—getting the correct data—it may be too much to ask them to let go. They unwittingly try to maintain tight control over the content of the interview. In contrast, an interviewer to whom a nondirective interview comes naturally feels comfortable in accepting the story as it comes from the patient. This, then, is what is meant by a nondirective interview: accept the patient's story as he or she wants to tell it. It means not directing the patient to give a story in the form or order that you want to receive it. Patients have problems, anxieties, and things they feel they need to tell. A nondirective approach allows them to tell what is on their minds.

Having accepted this, can the student expect all patients to know what they want to say? Is this whole business of interviewing just a matter of keeping one's mouth shut while the history unfolds, perhaps adding a few remarks to show interest? That would be good, but not all patients are that well-organized and sometimes they must be helped to discover what to explore. In the next chapter, I will discuss ways to help patients recognize what they want to explore. Is this another paradox? We show the patients how to discover what is best for them. I don't think so, but readers can make up their own minds. The interviewer should help the patient to explore areas that our best information and theory tell us are important determinants of behavior: current relationships, early psychosocial development and relationships, physical problems, and others. We help to point the patient in the direction where, to the best of our knowledge, explorations will be most productive, while allowing enough latitude to explore areas the doctor will inevitably miss.

Even though a good medical interview cannot be entirely nondirective—because certain information must be obtained—*begin* in the nondirective mode, because this sets the tone for the entire interaction. Too many questions too early in an initial interview confuse patients about what information is wanted, and they are discouraged about volunteering information. Patients can be confused because they are not yet certain what the doctor wants to hear. If the doctor frequently interrupts, he or she obviously doesn't want to hear what the patient is saying. Patients begin to wait and let the doctor tell them what to do. At this point the tone is set for an authoritarian (doctor)–submissive (patient) interview. Doctors are seen as authority figures and, although this cannot be completely eliminated, it should be minimized in the spirit of mutual exploration.

Starting with a general question that requires some thought on the part of the patient encourages exploration and does not lead to short, what we might call "terminating," answers. A terminating answer would be one that completes the information to be delivered and requires no additional response or thought from the patient. After a terminating answer, the patient can sit back and wait for the doctor to make the next move. "How old are you?" is such a question. We sometimes need to ask such questions, but it is better not to at the start of the interview. There are exceptions, as we shall see.

Helping the Patient to Start

How do we give patients permission to begin talking about whatever is on their minds as it relates to their problems? We want the patient to begin where he or she wants; not where the doctor thinks he or she should begin. There are many ways to do this and each person will eventually develop his or her own style. If it is in a clinic, one can say "Perhaps you can tell me what brings you in today." A patient, in responding to such a question, will usually begin by stating what he or she considers to be the most pressing problem. "I can't concentrate and I have no interest in the things I enjoyed in the past," for example.

Sometimes patients are reluctant to start talking or may even be angry about being interviewed. If patients say, "Because my doctor told me to come back," the interviewer must immediately wonder what feelings patients have to cause that response. Did they not want to come back? Are they angry with their doctor? Are they tired of seeing a new medical student? One might respond by saying, "Why did your doctor ask you to come back?" If the patient says, "I don't know," it may be that he or she doesn't want to, or can't, communicate. Instead, one could say, "How do you feel about coming back?" The first question is more factual; the second aims at the feelings behind the comment.

Which question to use is a matter of judgment and this judgment is based on knowledge and experience. The patient may be doing well and returning for a routine visit. If the physician thinks this is the case, then the first, more factual, question is appropriate. The doctor may, however, sense a high level of anger or other feelings. If so, the feeling question is more appropriate. Helping the patient express these feelings may remove barriers to future communication.

One question by the physician and one answer from the patient have already raised a multitude of questions in the doctor's mind. He or she is also faced with a number of decisions about what to say next and which directions to explore. I won't answer all of these questions, nor is there an unambiguous map that tells where to go, but I hope to make the decisions and the path easier.

After the patient knows the purpose of the interview, another way to start is to say something like, "Why don't you begin wherever you like?" This may be too much latitude for some, so when the reply is, "I just don't know where to begin—will you help me?" you can say, "Why don't you start by telling me about your daughter, Joan, who you brought to the clinic . . . is having trouble in school . . ." or whatever. If at all possible, try to stay away from questioning that requires one-word or short, definitive answers. Here is an example from a recorded interview. This is a continuation of one of the examples used in the second chapter.

> DOCTOR: Mr. A, I'd like to have you tell me a bit about what your problems have been through the years. You might start out by telling me how you got into the hospital.
>
> PATIENT: How I got into the hospital, I was drinking. I got divorced. I lost everything I had. I started drinking. I started taking dope and then I mixed them both together. I don't know what would happen, but I'd take off and walk. I could walk five days and it would just seem like one day. Just walking. (pause)
>
> DOCTOR: Then you would end up . . .? (A better comment might have been, "Sounds like you were having a bad time." This is

better because it is less specific but still helps the patient focus on what was going on at that time.)

PATIENT: No place. No goal or anything.

DOCTOR: You weren't going anyplace?

PATIENT: No, I wouldn't sleep, wouldn't eat. I'd be afraid inside, but I had a compulsion. Didn't know what I was going to do. I'd stay at a friend's house for a couple of days. Then I'd run away from there. I ran away from here once.

The amount of material presented in such a short time is bewildering. Each statement the patient makes raises more questions and none of these questions is yet answered. Just to mention a few:

How much does he drink? When did it start?

What does the divorce have to do with it?

What kind of dope?

What does he mean, five days were one day?

What does he remember during those five days?

Why not ask some of these questions? Because each specific question prompts the patient to think more narrowly. Early in the interview, it is better to avoid narrowing down. Rather, we should keep these questions in mind. They are important. The patient will probably answer them in due course. If not, we can always go back to fill in the gaps. I say this fully realizing that this method may offend the orderly sensibilities of some who prefer to complete one thing before going on to another.

Some patients are a little more anxious and uncertain, and the interviewer must talk with them more, put them at ease, and establish rapport before they will go ahead. In the following example, an anxious patient, while walking down the hall toward the interview room with the doctor, asked what the interview was about and what the doctor was going to want to know. It was apparent that the young man was not only frightened, but that he experienced the doctor as an authority who would tell him what to do. This patient had already relinquished control of the interview; that is, the patient said, "Tell me what you want." He was too anxious to think about what he would like to tell the doctor. This is what we are trying to avoid. You don't want the patient to sit waiting for questions; therefore, the first task in this interview is to give the initiative back to the patient so that the patient feels helped and not rejected.

DOCTOR: You asked if I could tell you ahead of time what questions I would ask. What I would like to do is to get some idea of your problems and how you have been living your life. How old are you?

This direct question seemingly violates the rule for a nondirective interview. It is a terminating question. It was put in partly to get necessary information, but more importantly to break up the doctor's monologue and allow the patient to say something and help to get the interaction going. It is easy to fall into a pattern of delivering monologues when a patient seems to have trouble talking. Watch out for them.

PATIENT: I'm nineteen.

DOCTOR: I would like to hear about what has been happening to you lately and how your early life has contributed to what is going on now. This is what I am interested in, so why don't you just start out. Start anyplace you want.

The patient now has the responsibility for a major share of the interview. The doctor has assumed his share of the responsibility by indicating what he is interested in, but he has clearly structured the interview as a cooperative endeavor.

PATIENT: Start lately? Well, lately I've been doing a lot of dope and stuff.

The patient is still leaning heavily on the doctor's authority and lead, but he is willing to give it a try. He would probably be more comfortable if he were asked direct questions. Direct questions might get answers to what was on the doctor's mind, but might not tell us what was on the patient's mind.

Some will find it difficult to return the responsibility for proceeding with the interview to the patient because this is contrary to our social training. We have been conditioned to answer questions and to help people. When a patient who is obviously frightened says, in effect, "Please help me and make me less frightened by asking me questions," we automatically respond by doing what the patient wants; otherwise, we feel guilty. It should relieve the student's guilt to realize that it is detrimental to encourage the patient to become overly dependent. The patients' interests are better served if they are stimulated to think about their problems. We should try not to allow patients to become so anxious that they are disorganized, but they may need to tolerate a reasonable amount of anxiety while taking responsibility for presenting their story.

Another reason that some students find it difficult to give the patient responsibility for beginning the interview is that this seems to be an abrogation of responsibility. When the patient says, "How do I start?" students feel guilty if they don't know and can't tell their patients how to start. Both the student and the patient have their guilts and anxieties to deal with as the relationship begins. Learning to deal with these feelings is part of learning to interview.

Once the patient begins, some reponse is required from the physician. If the patient keeps talking, the response need only be a show of interest. If the patient stops after a sentence or two (as patients frequently do) then the physician should make a comment. The comment must be sensitive to the patient's feelings and earlier statements and must encourage the patient to continue with what is on his or her mind. Before the doctor says anything, he or she must first choose from a number of possible statements. The course of the interview will hinge on these choices. This is illustrated in the next example, taken from a medical student's interview with a 68-year-old woman who had been seen in medicine clinics four times over the past one and one-half years.

STUDENT: How are you today? What seems to be the trouble?

PATIENT: Doctor, I just feel tired and run down all the time. My headaches have been getting worse and I just can't sleep at night. (Patient stops)

STUDENT: Why can't you sleep at night?

PATIENT: Well, doctor, I just am not sleepy. There is so much noise around my apartment that I'm continually upset. I think I have high blood pressure.

The response, "Why can't you sleep at night?" was logical, but it was not the correct response, because the patient did not elaborate on not sleeping. This lack of response means that she did not want to talk about not sleeping. To continue to dwell on this topic will not be productive, at least now.

STUDENT: Where are you living, ma'am?

PATIENT: I had to move into a low-rent housing project two years ago. My husband died six years ago and my children have been helping me less and less.

"Where are you living, ma'am?" was a good response. The patient picked up on it and is beginning to talk about what is on her mind. If the student does not stop her, everything will go smoothly. The patient's response to the doctor's question, statement, or nod of encouragement is one of the best indicators of whether or not the doctor did the right thing. A question or comment that brings forth important material from the patient is usually a good one. This is one criterion the interviewer uses to decide whether or not his or her reply to the patient was appropriate.

Those learning interviewing should at least try to keep in mind the immediate sequence of the doctor–patient interaction. The patient's response is often best understood in terms of the doctor's preceding remark. The problem is to learn how to make such a good response to a patient's comments. At first glance this may seem easy, but as with many other aspects of medicine, the more one studies the subject, the more one sees complicating questions.

Let's review the first statement made by this patient and analyze possible responses that the doctor could make.

> PATIENT: Doctor, I just feel *tired* and *run down all the time*. My *headaches* have been *getting worse* and I just *can't sleep at night*.

The words in italics emphasize the number of possibilities for response presented by the patient in her two short sentences. The student must choose what to say or say nothing, which is also a choice. Below are some possibilities. You can probably think of others.

> Tired?
>
> What do you mean "run down"?
>
> Where are your headaches located?
>
> Getting worse?
>
> Why can't you sleep?
>
> Go on.
>
> Say nothing.

A typical, but probably unproductive, response would be, "Where are your headaches located?" This question, meant to gather more specific information about a physical symptom, would probably stop the flow of information about the patient's life situation, and the latter appears to be most responsible for her symptoms. We need to know where her headaches are located, but we can and should return to this at a more appropriate point in the interview. Types of responses will be discussed in the next chapter.

A psychiatric interview differs somewhat here from a typical medical interview, although it should not differ as much as it sometimes does. Typically, a family practitioner or internist wants to know as much about the headache (where it radiates, and so on) as possible. So does the psychiatrist. The patient might have a brain tumor. Brain tumors cause deviant behavior, too. But the psychiatrist also wants the patient to express thoughts and feelings spontaneously. For this reason, the psychiatrist may postpone finding out about the headaches until later in the interview and thus avoid being too directive too early.

Some Problems with Directive Interviews

Directive interviewing has its place, but it can present problems, especially early in an interview. An interview that is started off in a directive manner tends to become more directive and less productive of spontaneous information as it progresses. The quality of the interview is often inversely related to the specificity of questions that the doctor asks early in the interview. The patient may talk quite a bit after each of the first few questions, but he or she will always pause and wait for the next question. Answers often become shorter and the physician must think fast to find another question.

We mentioned that direct questions set a different interview tone and mode for interacting. Here are some examples. The first interview is with a young couple who brought their baby to a neighborhood pediatric clinic. They are being interviewed before a small group of first-year medical students. The student is conducting his first interview in front of the group.

> STUDENT: I really appreciate your coming in here and giving us the opportunity to talk a little while. And why don't we start out, perhaps with you, Mr. R, and tell us about what you do and a little bit about yourself.
>
> PATIENT: I work in civil service. (pause)
>
> STUDENT: Civil service, you say?
>
> PATIENT: Yeah.
>
> STUDENT: What do you do in civil service?
>
> PATIENT: Right now I'm driving a truck.
>
> STUDENT: You what, sir?
>
> PATIENT: Driving a truck. (Patient talks rapidly in a low voice that is difficult to understand.)
>
> STUDENT: How long have you worked for the city?
>
> PATIENT: 'Bout two years.
>
> STUDENT: Two years?
>
> PATIENT: Yeah.
>
> STUDENT: And, uh, were you born here?
>
> PATIENT: Yes sir.

The interview continues in this way until it is terminated in about twenty minutes. Mr. R and his wife are being interviewed together and he is holding a six-week-old infant on his lap. The infant was brought to the clinic. The parents are both anxious and relatively nonverbal. The interview could probably not be "saved." By that we mean the parents could probably not be guided to talk spontaneously about themselves and their family; however, several approaches could have been tried.

If the student were not so anxious himself, he could have allowed the pauses to go on longer. Instead, each time there was even a short pause, the student, to relieve his own anxiety as much as anything else, would ask a question and thereby reinforce the authoritarian–submissive nature of the interview.

The student might have tried to engage Mr. R in more conversation about his work. Or he might have said, "I'm asking all of the questions here. Maybe there are other things on your mind that you would like to tell us."

When an interview becomes too directive, with too many requests from the doctor for specific facts, it becomes an interrogation. It is almost as if the room were dark, the spotlight on the patient, and the interrogator were saying, "Just give me the facts." In rare instances, interviewers lean so far in this direction that they attempt to trip the patient up.

The following is a segment of a directive interview taken verbatim from a videotape.

DOCTOR: Good afternoon, Ann.

PATIENT: Hi.

DOCTOR: Is this the first time you have come to the clinic?

PATIENT: Yes, it's my first time.

DOCTOR: How did you first find out about the clinic?

PATIENT: From school.

DOCTOR: Where the children go to school? The teacher?

PATIENT: The nurse.

DOCTOR: Aha, the nurse.

PATIENT: The nurse.

DOCTOR: What did she tell you?

PATIENT: They called me up and told me to bring my children over here to be checked.

DOCTOR: How many children do you have?

PATIENT: I've got three, two in school.

DOCTOR: And one at home?

PATIENT: Yes.

DOCTOR: Are you on welfare?

PATIENT: Yes.

DOCTOR: How old are you?

PATIENT: Twenty-seven.

DOCTOR: Twenty-seven. (pause) Are the children having any problems in school?

PATIENT: Well, my oldest son, he's having problems reading and they say he could be mentally retarded, but he's not. I've had him checked.

DOCTOR: Uh huh, he seems kind of small for his age. Is your husband small?

PATIENT: Yes, he's kind of small and skinny.

DOCTOR: How tall is he?

PATIENT: About five feet two.

DOCTOR: Are you living with your husband?

PATIENT: No, I've been separated four years from him.

DOCTOR: Where is your husband now?

PATIENT: He's out playing around.

DOCTOR: How do the children take to him? Does he come to see them?

PATIENT: No, they never see him. They see him once in a while, but hardly ever. They're not very close to him because he was in the penitentiary. He was there for about two years and a half and when he came out, we never got back together.

DOCTOR: He was in the pen for what?

PATIENT: For drugs. Burglary and drugs.

DOCTOR: And during that time did you work?

PATIENT: No, I was a housewife.

DOCTOR: Did you go on welfare?

PATIENT: Yes.

DOCTOR: How long has he been out?

PATIENT: About four years.

DOCTOR: When he came out, is that when you decided to separate?

PATIENT: We stayed together about two months, but didn't make it. We were fighting.

DOCTOR: Did he have another woman?

PATIENT: Yes.

DOCTOR: Have you been on drugs?

PATIENT: Yes. I guess I loved him so much that I wanted to be with him and find out how it was. Then he found this other girl.

DOCTOR: How did you start first? How do people first start?

On the surface this might appear to be a good interview because certain factual information was obtained. We learned that the patient is 27 years old. She has three children, one of whom is not doing well in school and may be retarded. She is on welfare and separated from a husband who is playing around and doesn't come to see her. We learn that the husband has been in prison and that they have both been on drugs.

Even though that much information has been obtained, the patient has assumed almost no responsibility for the interview. She has reacted to the interviewer by talking about each question, then stopping and waiting for the next question. Sooner or later, whether in the first interview or a subsequent one, the interviewer will run out of questions and the doctor–patient relationship will be difficult to maintain because the entire relationship was based on question and response. These unspoken, unwritten rules were set down by the doctor.

The interview has produced considerable information, but so far we know nothing about the woman who is experiencing the events. What are her hopes and fears? What is she feeling? Who is she? How does she feel about having a child who is small for his age? Does she reject him because he is like his father with whom she fights? In part, the doctor–patient relationship should be a controlled communication of feelings. This does not happen during a question and answer interview.

Contrast this with a third-year medical student's interview in a medical clinic, in which she learns how a patient's life situation contributes to the symptoms that bring the patient to the clinic. We first met this 68-year-old woman a few pages back when we were analyzing responses to initial statements:

STUDENT: How are you today? What seems to be the trouble?

PATIENT: Doctor, I just feel tired and run down all the time. My headaches have been getting worse and I just can't sleep at night.

STUDENT: Why can't you sleep at night?

PATIENT: Well, doctor, I just am not sleepy. There is so much noise around my apartment that I'm continually upset. I think I have high blood pressure.

STUDENT: Where are you living, ma'am?

PATIENT: I had to move into a low-rent housing project two years ago. My husband died six years ago and my children have been helping me less and less.

STUDENT: Would you describe your headaches, that is, how and when they occur and in what part of your head are they?

She should have encouraged the patient to talk about her situation, but here is an example of how a mistake does not ruin an interview.

PATIENT: It always starts in the back of the neck and goes completely over my head. They are always there, but are more severe in the late afternoon. I would also like to tell you about my leg aches, doctor. It is getting so that I can hardly walk. With my headaches and legs hurting, I just feel bad all the time. I never get any sleep either. I just feel worn out all the time.

STUDENT: Mrs. X, could you tell me something about your neighbors? (Here she gets back to the patient's worries.)

PATIENT: Oh, doctor! They are just awful. They drink all the time and have parties late at night. The children are always running through my flowerbed.

STUDENT: Do you think that this might have something to do with your being upset all the time, Mrs. X?

PATIENT: Well, I just don't know. I know that it didn't give me high blood pressure.

STUDENT: Did you feel well physically before you moved to your present home?

PATIENT: Oh yes, doctor. Why I never had a sick day in my life until I started coming to this hospital.

STUDENT: Was that before or after you moved?

PATIENT: Well, let's see; it was after.

STUDENT: Ma'am, you have a very common complaint, that is, about your headache.

PATIENT: Really, doctor, I was afraid I had cancer.

STUDENT: No, ma'am, you have what we call tension headaches and it is caused by the muscles in your head and neck being too tight. Have you noticed any relation between being or becoming anxious and the onset of your physical complaints?

PATIENT: No, I have never thought about it.

STUDENT: Have you felt well in the past six months?

PATIENT: Yes, when I visited my sister for two weeks. Doctor, are you really saying all my pains are in my mind?

STUDENT: No, not at all. I feel that all your pains are present just as you say they are. Now, Mrs. X, we have been over you physically several times and have run numerous tests. The tests have always been normal and we have never found anything physically wrong with you.

PATIENT: But one doctor told me I had high blood pressure. (Blood pressure of 140/95 was once recorded in the chart; on two other occasions the patient was normotensive.)

STUDENT: Ma'am, your blood pressure was at the upper limits of normal one time and has been normal on two other occasions. You definitely have normal blood pressure. Mrs. X, I would like for you to tell me truthfully how your home situation is affecting you.

PATIENT: Doctor, it just keeps me upset all the time and I do feel that if I could just get away I would feel better.

STUDENT: I feel the same way, Mrs. X. I think that you are becoming so anxious about these things that you are causing yourself these physical difficulties. I would like for you to think about these things we have talked about and try to become a little less anxious.

PATIENT: I will, doctor.

Student's summary: It became more and more evident to the patient during the conversation what her trouble was. She seemed very much relieved when I told her that nothing was wrong with her physically and that she didn't have hypertension. During the conversation she showed signs of becoming less and less anxious and she was talking freely and smiling at the conclusion. When she left she thanked me several times and said that I was the only doctor that had talked to her. I felt that this is the only patient that I have seen in medicine clinics that I have really gotten positive results that I could see.

The student may not have solved all this patient's problems or "cured" her illness, but she helped, through the discussion with her, as much as any medication. No doctor can "cure" all patients, but all doctors can, in some way, help all patients. The doctor–patient relationship itself can be therapeutic. What better example can we find than this?

This interview, although taken verbatim from the student's presentation, is not verbatim from the actual interview: therefore, the transitions seem a bit abrupt, more so than they actually were. The interview is more directive than it should be. It does not usually work as well to tell a patient that physical symptoms are caused by environment problems. But no interview is perfect, and this one well illustrates how a student in the middle of medical education is able to help many patients by letting them talk and express feelings.

The Opening Statement

The patient's opening statement tells the doctor how the patient wants to be viewed, what he or she wants to present, and something about how he or she will perceive the doctor–patient relationship. Listen carefully to the patient's first remarks. The opening statement is a behavioral synthesis of material from the unconscious and conscious mind. It gives a glimpse of hopes and fears from the deeper reaches of the mind and of how the doctor and the present situation are perceived. The patient's opening statement could stimulate many questions in the doctor's mind—questions to be filed for answers or further clarification later.

Listen to an opening statement. A patient from the psychiatric service volunteered to be interviewed by a medical student in front of a small group of other students. The student said, "Would you like to begin by telling us what brought you to the hospital?"

The patient answered, "I had blisters all over my feet. Got them from running with bad shoes, but the doctors didn't do anything for my feet. They are better now anyway."

The student was taken aback and said, "Is that all that brought you in?"

The patient smiled and said, "Well, my sister had me committed because she was afraid that I was going to get violent again with my father."

An important rule to remember is that *no* behavior is irrelevant or unimportant even if the meaning is not immediately apparent.

Why did this patient talk about his feet at this time? What did he want to tell us or conceal from us? We can't answer these questions now, but here are some important questions that the student should file in his or her mind to be examined and confirmed or refuted at a later date:

> Does he think we won't accept him if he has mental problems?
>
> Is he telling us that he is not receiving any help here in the hospital for his real problems? He said the doctors didn't treat his blisters.
>
> Maybe he thinks I won't understand his mental problems, but that I can relate to his physical problems.
>
> Is the statement symbolic of something else on his mind?

Early in the first interview, it is not appropriate to investigate all of these hypotheses, but it might be later. With these questions in mind the student can listen for other things the patient says about how his doctors treat him in the hospital.

Related to the opening statement is the question, "Why does the patient come in now?" This may seem like an absurd question when a patient who is obviously in distress presents for treatment. Yet time and again we find that many psychiatric and other medical problems have been long-standing. So, why does this patient come now rather than yesterday, or a week ago, or tomorrow? If this question can be answered—and it cannot always be answered—you will have important information about the patient's relationship to his or her environment, which is always a major element in psychiatric illness.

With some idea of how to begin, how to respond, and what to listen for, we can move now to the body of the interview.

Reference

Ries RK, Hunt DD, Ward NG, Mason JC: Medical students and psychiatric patients: an encounter of the first kind. *J Med Educ* 1980;55:773–777.

4

The Body of the Interview

Obtaining a Psychiatric History Using a Nondirective Approach

A good interview is a complex process that requires many decisions along the way. To conduct a proper interview, the physician must understand and be aware of as many of these complexities as possible. As I have already discussed, they result from the past history and feelings that both the doctor and patient bring to the interview. The doctor must skillfully use his or her knowledge and intuition to assist the patient constructively through this complex experience, to derive information, and to explore material that will be helpful to both doctor and patient.

Once the patient takes the lead in this exploration, the interview becomes a constructive, collaborative experience. The patient can give voice to feelings and learn more about his or her thoughts, fears, guilts, and ambitions while being guided to discuss areas about which the doctor must gain important information. At its best, the interview is an exciting adventure of discovery for the patient and doctor. Some patients become intrigued with this self-exploration. With these patients, you only have to show some interest in a particular area or something that the patient mentions to stimulate exploration into events in his or her past life. Here is an example that continues with Mr. A, whom we first met when discussing opening the interview. The patient is talking about his compulsion to run:

> DOCTOR: How long have you had a feeling like that? (running)
>
> PATIENT: Almost a year.
>
> DOCTOR: Can you remember when it started?
>
> PATIENT: Yeah, when I was working on the coast after that storm

(hurricane). I went down to work. There was no place to live. I couldn't get any water or electricity. I was sleeping in my wife's station wagon. I got panicky.

DOCTOR: You mean a feeling of fear inside?

PATIENT: It's not the kind of fear you get when someone pulls a gun on you. (He has had someone pull a gun on him.) It's a different kind of fear. It's hard to explain. It's inside you. After we were married and my wife would ask me to go to the store, I'd go down first and get a half pint and drink it. It sounds silly, at least it is silly to me now. (Patient pauses, not sure where to go, so the doctor steps in and encourages him to explore the roots of his fear.)

DOCTOR: As you say, it's an inside fear. Can you remember how long you have had this thing? It must have been with you since you were a little kid.

PATIENT: It must have been. You see, I lived in England during the war, World War II. (Patient begins to tie it together.) Mother was an alcoholic. She would be drunk when I would come home. (He then talks about his anger toward his mother when she came home drunk. He lived with her off and on through his teens.) When she'd be drunk and yell at me I wanted to beat her, but I couldn't. I would take it out on something else. (Then, when his wife asked for a divorce, he wanted to kill her. He had the same feelings toward her as he did toward his mother.)

DOCTOR: When you get angry. . . ?

PATIENT: I keep it inside me.

DOCTOR: You have to do something with it.

PATIENT: I usually go get drunk, take some pills.

During the next interview we learn more about how the past influences the present.

DOCTOR: I was particularly interested in your experiences in England.

PATIENT: You mean during the war?

DOCTOR: Yes, and as far back as you can remember.

PATIENT: I remember during the war planes being shot down and people being killed. I watched Madame Tussaud's burn down. You know, that wax museum.

DOCTOR: Must have been quite a fire.

PATIENT: Lot of candles. I was pretty much on my own over there. Mother worked.

DOCTOR: What was your first memory?

PATIENT: When I saw my father for the first and last time. (Father visited him when the patient was two years old, then returned to combat and was killed.)

The patient then discusses other times he felt deserted.

PATIENT: Mother went to work. My sister, she's three years older than me. She took care of me most of the time, when she felt like it.

DOCTOR: You seem to have some feelings about that.

PATIENT: We don't get along.

DOCTOR: Wonder how it feels to be on your own and running around a big place like London when you're six or seven years old.

PATIENT: It didn't bother me then. But it bothers me now. I hate to go downtown and I hate to be around people; but then it didn't bother me. Days are fine, but nights are rough. I want to take off running.

DOCTOR: Those are painful emotions.

PATIENT: They're not good feelings to have, but they didn't bother me until last year when they all started coming out. Why would they wait 'til then to come out?

DOCTOR: Any ideas? (Here most interviewers would be tempted to give an answer or an "interpretation.")

PATIENT: Maybe because my wife divorced me.

DOCTOR: How would that bring them out? Sounds like you have a hold of something there.

PATIENT: Well, like my mother would leave us and now she's (wife) gone, and that's when it got real bad.

DOCTOR: Brought out all that stuff?

PATIENT: Everyone needs a rubber duck—you know, something to cling to.

DOCTOR: What's your rubber duck? (Here one could say, What do you mean? but instead it is important to stay within the plan of the interview. Using the patient's own words helps.)

PATIENT: Ain't got one. Was my wife and kids. Anyone will tell you that—that you need a security blanket.

DOCTOR: And that was your wife. What was it before that?

PATIENT: I guess it was my mother. You see, I was living with my mother before I got married. Course I didn't enjoy staying with her, but I knew I had some place to go. It hits you kind of hard when you wake up one morning and it's . . .

DOCTOR: All over?

PATIENT: Yeah.

DOCTOR: Like out in the street again?

PATIENT: Like telling you you're not a doctor. Find yourself another job.

DOCTOR: Yeah, that would be pretty bad. Does it take away your identity?

PATIENT: Yeah.

This is an example of how a patient, with the help of the physician, can concurrently explore past history, present symptoms, and the relationship between the two. For the doctor to guide such an exploration, he or she must know and understand the influence of child development on present personality function. Doctors must be alert to the role of parents in early personality formation so that they can help the patient discuss this at the opportune time in the interview.

This is illustrated in a portion of the interview with the other young man we were discussing in "Opening the Interview":

PATIENT: My father was in the Army. We were stationed in England.

DOCTOR: I was interested . . . You hadn't mentioned your father until just this minute. You have talked about your sisters and your mother.

PATIENT: My father has always . . . we never have gotten along. He's always been one-sided. In arguments I've never been right. I just don't like to talk about it.

DOCTOR: You have a lot of strong feelings about him, then.

PATIENT: Yeah.

We needed to know about the relationship with his father, but waiting until the patient mentioned him allowed the interviewer to observe the patient's reluctance to discuss the topic. One can sometimes go through an entire psychiatric history in this way, without disrupting the patient's flow of thoughts and feelings. To do this properly, however, the doctor needs some kind of outline in his or her mind. He or she should not slavishly follow the outline but, rather, fill it in as patients tell their stories.

In all situations physicians must have an idea of what they need to know, but they must not let that overshadow what the patient wants to tell. Some students and some physicians, even those with long experience, will interrupt a patient who is giving important family information because that is not what the physician is interested in hearing at that time. When this happens, other important information that the patient was about to tell may be lost. The information may not again be forthcoming for a number of reasons. When patients are not allowed to tell their story as they want, they may get the message that their doctor doesn't want to hear about those problems. Patients are sensitive. They easily get this message. Or, patients may want to discuss something that is hard to talk about and can only muster their courage once. Because the physician has taken the lead in this situation, the patient perceives that he or she should wait to be led.

The doctor has interrupted the patient's associations and forced the patient onto another train of thought. This violates a cardinal rule: the doctor should not interrupt a patient's productive thoughts to satisfy his or her own needs. Not all that a patient has to say contributes to his or her own welfare or is necessary information. Some patients need to be interrupted, but this should be done with forethought and good judgment, certainly not to satisfy the interviewer's curiosity or need for information in a certain order.

This happens frequently when patients begin to discuss other areas before physicians feel they have enough detail about the present illness. For example, an interview with a narcotic addict was proceeding well. The patient had told about his present hospitalization and the drugs he had been taking just before being hospitalized. He talked about how he was a skilled craftsman and was earning enough money to support his habit without stealing. Then he said, "My father wanted me to go to college and I was smart enough, but I always wanted to do things my way." At this point the physician's need for order intervened: "Now just a minute. Can we go back? When was the first time you were in the hospital for this trouble?" How jarringly different this is from the statement, "You hadn't mentioned your father until just this minute."

It is important to know the time for first hospitalization, but not right then. A better statement, if any was needed, would have been "Tell me about that," or "Do things your way?" or "You seem to have some feelings about that," or something else to encourage the patient to say more about what is obviously bothering him. It would have been easy enough to come back another time and find out when the patient was first hospitalized.

In putting together a history, we are on an adventure of personal exploration where things will not always fall neatly into place nor will the meaning of things observed be immediately apparent. It is not an aimless exploration. Rather, it has a definite pattern and enough structure for us to recount where we have been. The ideal model for the exploration is one in which physician and patient play back and forth among present and past situations and problems in their effort to gain more information and further insight into the patient's current life, problems, success, deficiencies, and assets. This is a controlled exploration in which the physician must know the boundaries so that he or she may communicate to the patient some confidence that the journey will end happily rather than in disaster.

The interview with Mr. A illustrates this. We will analyze this interplay starting from the doctor's "Wonder how it feels to be on your own and running about a big place like London when you're six or seven years old?"

The patient responds, "It didn't bother me then, but it bothers me now. I hate to go downtown and I hate to be around people. . ."

Here we should hypothesize that he had intense fears as a 6-year-old, but was forced to deny them in order to survive. We don't say this to the patient, but the physician can't help but say to himself or herself, "Aha, his phobia started here." If we are so smart, why not share our intelligence with our patient? There are many reasons not to. First, we are not sure. Second, even if we are right, we are only partly right. Third, the doctor's insights do not necessarily help the patient. Finally, and most importantly, if we tell the patient and act as if we know it all, he or she will probably stop talking.

So, let's just encourage him and see what happens. The statement, "Those are painful emotions" allows him to go on. The patient agrees that they are not good feelings and says that they didn't bother him until last year. Then he asks, "Why would they wait 'til then to come out?"

Now the patient seems to ask for insight. Should we tell him? Are we being good doctors if we don't share what we think we know? Here the temptation to pontificate will be too much for some to resist. They will answer the patient, both doctor and patient will be relieved, and the exploration will stop, at least for a while.

Rather, let us choose to continue the exploration. The statement, "Any ideas?" accomplishes this. The patient now goes to work exploring his own mental processes. He says, "Maybe because my wife divorced me."

Again, the doctor makes an encouraging statement and the patient begins to link the feelings he had about his mother's leaving when he was small with those that he experienced when his wife left. "Well, like my mother would leave us and now she's (wife) gone and that's when it got real bad."

The doctor's next statement is another encouragement for the patient to go on and explore, but it is also a bit more. It approaches what we call an interpretation. That is, when the doctor says "Brought out all that stuff?" he is saying that the wife's leaving precipitated and brought out buried childhood feelings that first developed when the patient felt deserted by his mother and was forced to fend for himself. Notice that the doctor did not spell this out in detail to the patient. It wasn't necessary to do so and, furthermore, it would have stopped conversation. Don't pontificate too much.

The patient got the point, at least his unconscious did. We know this by his next response, "Everyone needs a rubber duck—you know, something to cling to."

Linus uses a blanket instead of a rubber duck. Some children have a teddy bear. One usually thinks of a child's security symbol as something warm and soft. A rubber duck sounds cold and a little hard. It may not be to this man but, on the other hand, it may be all the security he can muster.

He is talking about a fundamental need that, at best, has been only partially fulfilled in his life. Again, the doctor encourages him to explore this:

DOCTOR: What's your rubber duck?

PATIENT: Ain't got one. Was my wife and kids. Anyone can tell you that—that you need a security blanket.

DOCTOR: And that was your wife. What was it before that? (Here we are actively exploring the interplay among present, immediate past, and distant past: the developmental approach.)

PATIENT: I guess it was my mother. (Again we are on the right track. More information and more feelings come out.) You see, I was living with my mother before I got married. Course I didn't enjoy staying with her . . .

It turns out that not only did the patient feel deserted by his mother when he was a young child, but she was also an alcoholic who provided heartache and conflict for the patient when he was living with her before he married.

The trauma of living through a severe hurricane and, shortly thereafter, losing his last semblance of a "security blanket," his wife, brought forth with great force the earlier feelings that he had repressed and denied as he grew up.

This shows how an interview can explore present and past, moving from one to another to make relationships. At times, the process may appear haphazard and disorderly. We are always tempted to clean it up. But beware, the unconscious is not always neat. We should remember that many great archeological finds are made rummaging through the buried trash heaps of ruined cities. Much of the patient's insight comes in the emerging relationships of one buried item to another. Archeologists have some knowledge of ancient civilizations, and their digging is more organized than it may first appear. So it is with psychiatrists.

The patient we have been discussing gets "panicky." When his wife sends him to the store, he had to relieve his fear with a few drinks. He may have a panic disorder, which is often alleviated by medication. Even if he has a diagnosable mental disorder for which we can prescribe medication, it does not relieve us of the responsibility to help him explore past and present psychosocial events which contribute to his present problems.

Adding Structure

We have already stated that an important function of a medical interview, whether it be in psychiatry, family practice, internal medicine, or other specialties, is to gather needed and, for certain aspects of the problem, detailed information. An entirely open-ended approach to interviewing will not accomplish this *and* obtain all of the needed information we have discussed. As the interview progresses some parts must be more structured. This structure is compatible with the approach we have been describing providing it is used properly and with timing which is best suited to the patient.

Starting with an open-ended approach allows the patient to get his or her point of view across and, as we have discussed in detail, allows for the development of the history in the patient's own way. Encouragement to explore relevant areas is given in many ways both verbally and nonverbally. By expression of empathy and understanding, and sometimes direct questions, feelings are encouraged. Specific lines of questioning may also be used at various times in the interview and near the end to gather detailed information about specific areas.

The more structured part of the interview has become increasingly important in psychiatry as diagnosis becomes more exacting and more specific treatments are discovered. Panic disorders and manic and depressive disorders are examples of this. To establish whether or not these disorders are present, one must make inquiries into a number of areas of a person's life and ask about specific symptoms. Structured interviews have been developed for research protocols so that diagnoses can be comparable from one study to another.

Cox, Hopkinson, and Rutter (1981) made both controlled and naturalistic studies using different prescribed interview styles to determine which styles elicited the most information, which styles were more likely to elicit feelings and which may elicit both. In both naturalistic and experimental interviews, all of which were recorded on videotape and carefully studied, the authors confirmed the value of an open-ended interview combined with carefully chosen probes or questions. In their study, those interviewed were mothers who brought their children to a psychiatric clinic. The mothers who talked more gave more information, and there was a striking reciprocal relationship between the mother's utterances and the talkativeness and directiveness of the interviewer. The more the interviewer talked, the less the mothers talked. Here is direct evidence that an intrusive, directive style inhibits spontaneous talk.

The more the mothers talked, the more likely they were to give information about pathology and about important feelings. Mothers who were encouraged to express their concerns in their own way mention almost (but not quite) as many problems as when systematic questioning of an active type is employed. Feelings are also more likely to be expressed with interview styles that are less probing. More directive interview styles elicit the absence of pathology—that is, normality that mothers do not tend to mention.

On the other hand, direct questions and probes have a definite place in the interview. When interviewers were sensitive and alert to factual data and carefully probed for it, then more detailed information was obtained. Furthermore, the use of direct probes at specific times was not incompatible with the open-ended approach and could be combined with methods used to encourage the expression of feelings. Once an area is opened up in ways we have suggested, the directive questions can give good data about frequency, duration, and quality of symptoms.

Cox and colleagues also found that some patients were not forthcoming unless they were given more structure and more direct questions in the beginning. It is important that this structure not be in the form of closed questions because these do not encourage the free expression of feelings.

A combined structured and nonstructured interview approach was used in a study of marijuana users (Haas et al 1987). The authors found that the two approaches complemented each other. The structured approach could produce a comprehensive picture of actual behavior as well as consciously held thoughts and beliefs. The unstructured approach could uncover motivations and other information not otherwise consciously available. For example, the subjects, in response to structured questions, indicated that they smoked marijuana "to get pleasure, to feel good, to get high." The intensive, unstructured psychodynamic approach revealed "how hard pleasure came to most of these individuals." The material revealed in the psychodynamic interviews placed the material obtained from the structured interviews in a context that would not otherwise have been possible. These authors used the structured approach prior to using the more unstructured psychodynamic approach. This was part of the experimental design and not the best suited to the development of the doctor–patient relationship.

The types of structured interviews used for research have been found to adequately gather data on symptoms and the diagnosis that depends on them, but have serious limitations in the comprehensive overall evaluation of an individual (Carpenter et al 1976).

In moving from the nondirective to the more directive areas of the interview, it is important to be aware of the amount of authority assumed by the doctor as opposed to giving the patient more responsibility for the interview. As the doctor uses more direct questions, it is easy to slip into the role of the authority figure and for the patient to assume a more passive role. Many patients will assume this role easily and consequently relinquish responsibility for exploration and treatment of their problem.

Several authors have studied the relative authoritarian position of the doctor in relationship to the patient. Byrne and Long studied this in a general medical setting, and they developed a classification of behavior along a continuum of patient-centered/doctor-centered (Binjs et al 1984). In their study, they found that doctors tended to use a more patient-centered approach during the evaluation phase and then rapidly switched to the doctor-centered approach once they had made up their minds about diagnosis and treatment. As in the previously cited studies, the doctor's style had a definite effect on the patient's productions.

In a project undertaken by the Division of Primary Care and Family Medicine of the Harvard Medical School, Barsky and colleagues (1980) developed criteria with which to evaluate doctor–patient relationships in primary care. Some of the criteria they developed are as follows: "The physician should use the least amount of control, direction and activity necessary. This emphasizes the patient's role as an active and independent partner in the medical care process. . . . Insofar as is possible, the physician's authority should be limited to suggesting appropriate topics for the patient to address rather than asking specific questions."

Some Techniques

After having presented the general approach to interviewing and the importance to the doctor–patient relationship, we can now be more specific about techniques used to facilitate the interview. Techniques are not the interview, but rather specific ways to enable the interview to progress in the manner we have discussed.

The *open-ended question* is a technique and, as the reader may already have observed, there are degrees of open-endedness. "Tell me about yourself" is more open-ended than "Tell me what brought you to the hospital." "I'd like to know something about your past life" is more open-ended than "What was it like when you were growing up?" which, in turn, is more open-ended than "Can you tell me something about your mother?" All of these allow the patient to say what he or she wants, but some are more focused than others.

Focusing is another technique that allows for the development of more detailed information. Focusing is just what it says, bringing a part of the broader field into sharper definition. After a patient begins discussing an important topic area, there are often opportunities to ask more focused questions that will help to better evaluate the patient or help the patient to better understand the problem. For example, if a patient says she has no energy, you might ask, "Have you been feeling blue (or depressed)?" If the patient says yes, then the examiner would want to focus in more to find out how depressed the patient was and if there were suicidal thoughts. If there were suicidal thoughts, were there plans for suicide, which again narrows the focus.

As with all interviewing techniques, focusing is not done routinely, but must be used in the context of the total interview. Sometimes focusing will interrupt an otherwise productive discussion by the patient. If so, getting further details should be left to later in the interview.

A simple technique is *repeating the last words or phrase* that the patient has said. This shows interest in what the patient is saying, shows that the interviewer is listening attentively, and encourages the patient to go on with the topic being discussed. If a patient says, "I have been working hard lately" and then pauses, the interviewer could say, "What have you been doing?" or the interviewer could say, "Working hard?" Repeating the last word or phrase when used within the flow of the interview can keep the interview moving along. Longer questions may be more disruptive.

A technique used to encourage the discussion of feelings is called *reflecting*. This is commenting on the patient's feelings as they are observed in the interview. If the patient appears sad when talking about a depressing subject, the interviewer might say, "You look sad" or "That seems to make you sad." This encourages further discussion of the feelings and shows empathy on the part of the doctor. This often helps in the development of the doctor–patient relationship.

Clarification is often used to help understand what a patient is trying to say. It differs from focusing which gradually narrows the area of inquiry so that more detailed information may be obtained. Clarification is used to help the interviewer understand a complicated set of events or it may be used to help both patient and interviewer understand feelings and motivation.

A patient called eagerly requesting an appointment. When he came to the office, he said he had been depressed and thought that psychotherapy would help. During the interview he told of the books about psychology that he had been reading and about some self-help material that had greatly benefitted him. He had undergone therapy in the past and was not sure how much more he needed. Even though he initially said that he wanted psychotherapy, as the interview progressed it was apparent that he had some doubts about entering into therapy. This, then, required some clarification, which could begin in a number of ways. "You say you want therapy, but you also express some doubts about it." Or, "I'm not certain just what you are asking for."

Confrontation has some of the characteristics of clarification, but, in addition, it is an attempt to help the patient face something he or she may be reluctant to acknowledge. An alcoholic may say that he understands he has a problem and that he wants to quit drinking, so he is going to limit himself to one beer a night. The doctor might choose to confront him with the fact that this has not worked in the past and ask why the patient thinks it will work now.

Confrontation is useful to help the doctor judge the patient's insight and it is often helpful for the patient to understand inconsistencies and self-defeating behavior. Confrontation must be used with care, however, because it has the potential to disrupt the doctor–patient relationship. The patient may be forced too soon to see something that is being denied, or the doctor may confront in such a way as to appear hostile to the patient.

Specific techniques are useful during the course of the interview, but they are never a substitute for a collaborative doctor–patient relationship, which includes empathy with the patient. Specific techniques can, however, remedy some of the deficiencies commonly found in medical interviews. Maguire and Rutter (1976) studied videotapes of 15-minute interviews conducted by medical students to obtain a history on patients that they had never seen before. More than one third of the students avoided asking questions about personal issues. Most of the students did not find out what the patients meant when they said that they were run down or depressed, and most of the students did not pick up on verbal cues such as when a patient said "I was feeling low." To pick up on such a cue, the student would merely have had to repeat the last few words—"Feeling low?"

Outline for Psychiatric History

Harry Stack Sullivan said that the interviewer must always have in mind one question about the patient: "'Who is this person and how did he come to be here?' The generic answer is that a combination of his native endowments and personal experience has brought him to this pass'' (Sullivan 1954).

The following is a broad sweep of what to look for in a psychiatric history. The interviewer does not attempt to obtain this information in the order outlined or at one sitting. The topic outline recognizes the interplay of biological, psychological, and social forces in the etiology of mental illness. It also suggests that information obtained in these three areas be organized developmentally. This ideal cannot always be achieved, but we hope to stimulate thinking in developmental terms.

I.   Identification and demographic information
    A.   Name, address, phone number
    B.   Age
    C.   Sex
    D.   Place of birth
    E.   Marital status
    F.   Ethnic group
    G.   Occupation
    H.   Education

II. Present illness
    A.   Presenting complaint, problem, or problems
    B.   Onset, course, and duration
    C.   Events temporally associated with onset, exacerbation, and remissions
        1.   Other medical problems
        2.   Socioeconomic problems
        3.   Problems with interpersonal relationships
        4.   School or work situation
    D.   Developmental period associated with onset
    E.   Personality changes prior to or at onset of illness
    F.   Change in feelings about important people
    G.   Special things to look for: changes in eating habits, interests, routines, sleep patterns, feelings about work
    H.   Why does the patient come now?
    I.   Past and present treatments and treatment results

III. Medical history
    A.   Other current medical problems
    B.   Past medical history
    C.   Drug history
    D.   Systems review
    E.   Family medical history and history of mental illness, alcoholism, deviant behavior, etc.

IV. Psychosocial history—significant interpersonal relationships, feelings, and significant events from birth to present

A. Infancy
1. Circumstances surrounding birth
2. Relationship of mother and father
3. Socioeconomic situation of the family
4. Health of the mother and father
5. Principal caretaker or mothering figure

B. Toddler and preschool phase
1. Developmental milestones—walking, talking
2. Significant family events
3. New siblings
4. First memories

C. Middle childhood
1. School
a. Intelligence and successes and failures in school work
b. Problems with teachers
c. Other school-related activities
2. Peer relationships
3. Family relationships
4. Other activities
5. Physical growth

D. Adolescence
1. Peer relationships
2. Relationships with opposite sex
3. School
a. Academic
b. Other activities
4. Relationships with parents
5. Aspirations
6. Successes and failures
7. First use of alcohol and drugs

E. Adulthood
1. Work
2. Social relations
3. Sexuality and marriage
4. Family relationships
5. Economic circumstances
6. Changes with increasing age
7. Alcohol and drug use

F. Outlook and plans for the future in family, work, and social relationships

Throughout the entire history it is important to understand the patient's feelings about significant interpersonal relationships. These feelings may lend particular importance to the relationships. As an individual has only a limited number of such relationships, the task of understanding them is finite. Losses of significant personal relationships and the period of life when they occurred are especially important.

Identifying and demographic information must be obtained from all patients. This is usually noted on the medical record before the patient is interviewed; if not, it should be obtained during the interview. Sometimes the patient's anxiety can be relieved while obtaining this identifying information. The clinician says "Before we start, I'd like to get some specific information from you" and asks about age, marital status, and so on. This separates the early direct questioning from the later, more open-ended, interview.

The presenting complaint is foremost in the patient's mind and he or she is usually ready to explore it. Although I recommend that note-taking be kept to a minimum to avoid intruding on the developing doctor–patient relationship, it is useful to record the presenting complaint in the patient's own words. Using those words for the presenting complaint and occasionally as the history is recorded on the chart helps to capture individual nuances and character.

The present illness should be explored in as much detail as possible within the context of an open-ended interview and an empathic doctor–patient relationship. We need to know what was going on in the patient's life at the onset of the present illness. This includes a period before the stated onset of the illness, when there may have been other more subtle personality changes. Any physical illness or problems around the onset of the present illness are also important. They could be secondary to the psychiatric problems or of etiologic significance. Any environmental or interpersonal events should be explored as possible precipitating events.

Personality changes often precede the patient's version of when the present illness began. Changes in feelings about people or in patterns of sleeping and eating may also be early indicators of problems. The patient's illness may not have begun when, for example, he or she started having anxiety attacks in the elevator. It may have started with a job promotion and greater responsibility. That he or she now has an office on a higher floor and thus a longer elevator ride is only symbolic of underlying problems.

We often find that the presenting symptoms or problems have been present for a long time. Why does the patient come now? The interviewer should always ask this question. You will sometimes hear an answer something like this: "My wife said she would leave me if I didn't do something about my drinking." This alerts the interviewer to explore further the patient's motivation for treatment.

Before any treatment is begun, we must know what treatments the patient has had in the past and their results. These include organic, pharmacological, psychological, and social therapies. One medication may have been better than others, or perhaps a patient was improving with psychotherapy but was unable to continue for financial reasons. One must ask specifically about previous therapies. Patients do not usually volunteer this information.

A complete medical history and systems review is done so that other illnesses are not overlooked and because physical problems often contribute to mental illness. A history of drugs that have been taken will allow you to consider how they may be contributing to symptoms. Both prescribed and street drugs affect cognition and emotions. Occasionally we find that the entire psychiatric problem is due to the interaction of medication prescribed by one or more physicians.

Family medical history assumes more importance as we learn that certain mental illnesses may be genetically determined. The interviewer should ask about mental illness, alcoholism, and any other behavior or personality problems of family members. Parents' medical problems may at least have some psychological impact on children.

The next section, "The Importance of Childhood History," shows how information from the psychosocial history may be used in understanding the patient's problems. Information about early childhood may not be readily forthcoming. Patients may have repressed much of it. One way to begin to obtain past history is to say, "I'd like to know something about your past life. Why don't you start by telling me the first thing you can remember." Later in the interview, after memory is stimulated, the patient may recount even earlier memories.

When a patient is talking about past life experiences, the interviewer should try to picture how the events, relationships, or whatever the patient talks about may have been perceived by the patient when these events were experienced. A four-year-old may view the loss of a parent as punishment for bad thoughts. An adult will grieve, but he or she understands and accepts it without feeling responsible. A child, on the other hand, will interpret life events in terms of current developmental struggles. The patient talking about her past, in the chapter on psychotherapy (chapter 13), gives a dramatic example of how a young child interprets events differently from an adult.

Just as we want to know how a patient perceives the past, we also want to know about his or her outlook for the future. This question, "How does the future look to you?" can be surprisingly informative.

A seemingly realistic patient may have grandiose expectations of future successes. Other patients are content with a relatively bland future outlook. A depressed patient's view of the future is one measure of the extent of his or her depression.

The Importance of Childhood History

In psychiatry, in order to understand present illness it is essential to understand childhood history and past significant interpersonal relationships. To attempt otherwise would be like trying to understand the murmur of a patent ductus arteriosus without a knowledge of embryology.

Since ancient times we have known that experience during childhood has an influence on the formation of the personality; however, the subject has only recently been studied scientifically. Much is to be learned and some of what we think we know will undoubtedly prove to be incorrect. Yet we have learned some startling things. For example, children severely deprived of a maternal relationship during the first year of life may be mentally retarded and will be unable to form a stable relationship during the rest of their lives. Some will die in infancy, even if their nutritional and other physical needs are met.

Children from poor or lower class families with no intellectual stimulation before the age of six will often be slow learners in school and will be labeled mentally retarded. However, they would not have been retarded if they had had a different early childhood experience.

Violence also has its roots in childhood. Children who are beaten by their parents end up beating others and beating their own children. We often see a direct correlation between the amount of violence experienced by a child and the amount of physical violence delivered to others when he or she becomes an adult.

Most adult behavior is not as extreme and we must look for more subtle relationships between past experience and present behavior.

In the second chapter I gave the example of a patient whose perceptions began to approximate reality after successful psychotherapy. She thought that everything that happened to her was someone else's fault. Her mother died of cancer when the patient was four years old and within six months her father remarried. The patient, as a child, wanted desperately to please her new stepmother. Unwittingly, she began to take on the characteristics of the stepmother to identify with her. As an adult, the patient had two personalities. One was a proper lady with conservative manners who always had her hair fixed well. The other was a more relaxed, easy going, somewhat seductive woman.

For no apparent reason, the patient's personality would change abruptly from one interview to the next. The patient was aware of the change but could offer no explanation for it. During psychotherapy she became aware that the proper lady with the correct hairdo was her stepmother and this was her attempt to please the stepmother by being like her. A childhood need at the time of emotional trauma was repressed, but its derivatives persisted. We will learn more about this patient later.

The interplay of past and current experience in the formation of personality is complex and not yet completely understood. There are, however, some useful concepts in understanding this complicated interaction. The first is that of *regression*. A child or an adult, when faced with an overwhelming situation, regresses to an earlier mode of behavior. Doctors observe this time and again in most sick people. When faced with the fear and anxiety of illness, patients display some of the characteristics of earlier life periods. Depending on earlier life patterns they may be more demanding, more withdrawn, or more hostile and rebellious. A few people feel guilty about wanting to be taken care of, others are frightened by the idea. The latter may act overly independent to avoid the feared regression.

Another useful concept is that of *repression*. A traumatic experience or series of experiences in childhood is buried in the far reaches of the mind and, from then on, anything that reminds a person of the original experience brings forth the original childhood emotions attached to the experience. As long as the childhood trauma remains buried, it retains its childhood emotions and is not modified by later experience. The childhood emotions then transfer to present situations that may represent the original experience. This is one explanation of feelings and behavior that seem to be irrational. This phenomenon occurs in all of us, but most people are unaware of it. One goal of psychotherapy is to bring these experiences to light so that they may then be modified by a more mature intelligence.

When Mr. A (the patient we presented earlier) said it did not bother him to go out on the streets of London when he was little, but that now he hates to go downtown and to be around people, he is giving an example of this persistent childlike thinking. His repressed childhood fear is coming out in an inappropriate present situation. The terror of a young child alone in a war-torn city is now attached where it does not belong: to going downtown. The fact that we might diagnose a panic disorder in this patient, as we discussed earlier, does not negate the importance of these fears from early childhood.

Learning theory is also helpful in understanding this complicated interaction. Most simply stated, behavior that is rewarded is retained and that which is not rewarded, or is punished, is extinguished. If children are punished when they tell the truth, then they may soon learn to lie to avoid punishment.

These concepts help to bring some sense out of chaos, but nothing is quite as simple as it looks. We need only remind ourselves that some people get pleasure from punishment, which they seek over and over again, and others survive a traumatic childhood with few blemishes on a mature personality. The following brief examples illustrate how the knowledge of childhood experience helps us to understand what is happening now.

A 32-year-old man entered a Veterans Administration hospital with feelings of depression so severe that he was threatening suicide. He had been hospitalized twice before because of depression and feelings that people were against him. He also had attacks of rage and had beaten his wife on several occasions. She finally left him because of this.

He said he was doing well until he entered the service and was sent to Vietnam. There he built frontline fortifications and was frequently in the forefront of fighting. After this he became nervous and had nightmares. When he returned, he found out that his wife had been having an affair and his rage erupted.

After learning that he did well in high school—he was a track star and had many friends—I was tempted to say that the Vietnam experience was the major cause of his trouble, as it may indeed have been; however, as he talked more about his childhood, I learned that his father was stern and frequently used severe physical punishment. The patient was the one of his seven siblings most frequently and severely beaten by his father. Furthermore, he was close to his mother, who was loving and is still interested in him.

With this information about his relationship with his parents as he was growing up, I can no longer simply say that the fear and hostility created during the war caused his subsequent maladjustment. I learned more about the formation of his personality and the substrate on which the war experience might play.

We have spoken about how children who are beaten become violent adults. Some adults who experienced hostility as they were growing up can keep their hostility under control unless something provokes it or their control is weakened. With this patient, his controls were loosened in Vietnam and his rage provoked by an unfaithful wife. We can understand his feelings about fighting in Vietnam and then returning to find adultery in his home, but we must know his past childhood experiences to understand the depths of his hostility and despair. Furthermore, knowing what happened to him during childhood helps us to understand why he chooses a particular way of reacting.

Which, of all of these factors, is the major cause of this man's problems, or is there a single cause? I will leave aspiring young psychiatrists to ponder this and perhaps to carry out more definitive research in the future.

We know that the basic drives or instincts are always at work and somehow underlie all behavior: hunger, security needs, sexuality, territoriality, assertiveness, and mastery. They all play a role. Some are more prominent in one developmental stage than another. Patients whose childlike behavior is tied to a particular developmental stage that they never grew out of will prominently display an overabundance of the needs of that period.

The following illustrates this as well as how one explores problems in the present and recent past with a patient.

A 23-year-old man was brought to the hospital by his wife and mother because he was talking to his deceased father and father-in-law. He was depressed, unable to work, and complained of low back pain. During the first 30 minutes of the interview, he told of his visions and conversations with those who had died, his feelings that people were talking about him when he was in a crowd, and his drinking problem, which had started when he was in the Navy. He could tell his dead father his troubles and the father would console him.

It was not until the psychiatrist asked, "How were things while you were growing up?" that an understanding of his problem began to emerge. He said that life was rough. His mother and father were separated when he was four, after which his mother lived with a series of boyfriends. Several of them would beat her and the patient witnessed the beatings. The mother, in turn, would take out her frustrations by beating the children. As the patient grew older, he became more enraged. He once bought a gun to shoot one of his mother's boyfriends if he ever came around again. His mother found the gun, but not the bullets. She beat the patient until he found them for her.

He rarely, and only briefly, saw his real father during this time. When the patient was about 19, he and his father developed a closer relationship. The patient said, "He was understanding and gave me attention and many things. He tried to cram what he should have done all of the years we were growing up into those three years before he died."

One open-ended question was all that was needed to bring forth the information necessary to begin to understand the patient's life and the dynamics of his symptoms. But, if the psychiatrist did not have in mind an outline of what he needed to know, this childhood history might never have come to light. The patient's diagnosis was schizophrenia, but whatever it may have turned out to be and whatever the biologic substrate of the disease may be, the patient, as a person with his special symptoms, could only be understood through a knowledge of his early life history.

A 26-year-old man came to the hospital tired and bedraggled. His clothes were dirty. He was sunburned, dehydrated, and his feet were sore and swollen. He had been walking and hitchhiking from California to Texas. He was on his way to British Honduras to join its army. He was convinced that the country was soon to be invaded by the Russians. He occasionally had hallucinations. He would hear his old Army buddy urging him to go fight.

After two weeks of hospitalization and therapy with antipsychotic medication, he was much more lucid and able to tell of his past life. His father had been in the service and the family moved often. Until he was about 13, the longest they had stayed in one place was two and a half years. His father was away from home much of the time and the patient was close to his mother. When he was 14, his mother became ill and was in a coma for about a year. He went to the hospital every day to see her, but he said. "I was never able to bring her back."

He joined the Army before completing his senior year in high school and was sent to Vietnam. He was in the midst of fighting when he was hospitalized the first time.

Here again is a patient whose acute psychotic symptoms can be controlled by medication, but to better appreciate the pattern of his life one must understand his nomadic early life and relationship with his mother.

Keeping an outline of needed information in one's mind allows the interviewer to gather childhood and other historical material during an essentially nondirective interview in which it is the patient who determines the route and rate of exploration. Sometimes, however, the patient will halt the progress and you must detour. A man was talking about how his sister had him committed because she was afraid he was going to get violent again. He had thrown his father's cigarettes out of the house, all in fun, of course. After telling this, he pauses. The interviewer asks about trouble with the father and the patient says no more. Since he clearly, at least for now, does not want to express any more feelings about his father, the interviewer should return to some less emotionally laden subject. At such a point in the interview, asking for specific information will relieve tension while maintaining the flow of discussion. This, then, is one place in the interview to begin to fill in the outline with the necessary factual data for the psychiatric history. One could ask the patient how many brothers and sisters he has and how he ranks in age among them. Getting this information takes a short time. Asking about siblings is still in keeping with a subject that the patient has spoken about and it could lead to more discussion of how he feels about his siblings. If talking about siblings is not productive, one can easily return to the events surrounding the present illness with an open-ended question such as, "How were things going at home just before you came to the hospital?"

With experience, the interviewer should become adept at recognizing places in an interview where a specific question will not only yield important information, but will also serve an important function in the process of the interview. Eventually, every response, every statement, every action by the interviewer, will have a purpose and will benefit the diagnostic and the therapeutic function of the interview.

Feelings

Feelings are a particularly human characteristic and are magnificent when they are pleasant, but are especially uncomfortable for all when they are unpleasant. Feelings are not usually openly expressed or acknowledged in our culture. All cultures have prescribed ways of handling them, which children learn at an early age. For example, crying is expected at weddings and funerals, but may be accepted less well in other situations.

A number of mental mechanisms deal with upsetting feelings or those one may not want to express at the moment. A discussion of these mechanisms may be found in psychiatric texts. It helps to know these mechanisms because a psychiatric interview must explore feelings, and unpleasant feelings may be especially troublesome for the patient and the interviewer. People may try to handle unpleasant feelings by ignoring them. There are conscious and unconscious ways to ignore. For example, we repress unconsciously and sometimes display the feeling opposite to that repressed. This is called *reaction formation*. The patient who fears he may have a carcinoma of the lung because his smoker's cough is getting worse comes in to see his internist, with whom he has not made contact for five years, and says, "It's so good to see you, doctor." When he leaves, he says, "I hope we can visit more often." He is repressing the fear of seeing the doctor and of the possible carcinoma and is expressing the opposite reaction. Many other defense mechanisms are used to handle feelings, and most operate at an unconscious level. That is, the person is not aware, or only partially aware, of the feelings he or she is defending against. Sometimes it is hard to accept that a person is unaware of a feeling that is obvious to everyone around. A man may clench his fists, become red in the face, and say, "I'm not angry." He may be telling the truth and not be aware that he is angry even though he shows all the physiological signs of anger.

Being aware of the feelings but choosing not to display or mention them, is called *suppression*. This happens often, and appropriately so, in everyday contacts. But the doctor–patient relationship is not an everyday contact. It is special and carries with it special responsibilities on the part of the doctor and the patient. One of these responsibilities is to deal with feelings if they relate to illness or some problem the patient brings to the doctor.

Beginning interviewers have a tendency to avoid painful feelings if they threaten to come up in the interview. This is often done by changing the subject, and the interviewer not being aware that he or she is doing this.

SOME RULES ABOUT DEALING WITH FEELINGS

1. As much as possible, the interviewer should be aware of feelings in himself or herself and the patient.
2. Feelings are not always acknowledged.
3. Feelings are acknowledged when doing so will be helpful to the patient.
4. Feelings are usually acknowledged when they cause problems.
5. Feelings are usually acknowledged when that is supportive to the patient.
6. The doctor rarely, and then only carefully and with much forethought, discloses his or her own feelings to the patient.
7. Occasionally a patient may need help in maintaining control of his or her emotions.

1. *As much as possible, the interviewer should be aware of feelings in himself or herself and the patient.* This has been discussed in some detail in the chapter on the doctor–patient relationship.

2. *Feelings are not always acknowledged.* Although Rule 1 always applies, it does not follow that the doctor should comment on every feeling that he or she perceives in the patient. Some things are best left unsaid. Furthermore, commenting on every feeling may disrupt the flow of the interview.

Any statement made to the patient should have a purpose. Idle chatter is fine in a social situation, but it has no place in a doctor–patient relationship. The talk may appear to be idle, but for the doctor it should have a purpose. Lest this statement be misinterpreted, I am not saying that every statement must be serious and grim. Rather, there should be a rational and considered reason behind everything the doctor does. With knowledge of forethought, it is sometimes beneficial to discuss current fashions, or hunting, or fishing, or to joke with a patient. This may be done for a number of reasons: to relieve tension, to improve the relationship, to help the patient, to help the patient become aware that the physician, too, is a person. Whatever the purpose, it should be a considered act rather than a spontaneous or irrational impulse.

3. *Feelings are acknowledged when doing so will be helpful to the patient.* Patients benefit from permission to express anxieties, fears, and worries. In the first psychiatric interview with a patient, one might say, "You look pretty scared" if, of course, the person does look scared. Or, to the patient who comes in with chest pain, the doctor might say, "I'll bet you have been pretty worried about what might be going on to cause that pain." These remarks let the patient know that it is all right to have such feelings and to talk about them. Sometimes a statement such as "Want to tell me about it?" should be added to the acknowledgment of the feelings.

4. *Feelings are usually acknowledged when they cause problems.* Fear, anxiety, and hostility can frequently cause problems that impede the progress of the doctor–patient relationship. We have already commented on anxiety. Hostility is seen more often than one might suspect. A person may be angry at being sick or dependent. Intense anger is related to many psychiatric problems.

Sometimes a patient's angry feelings will block any attempt to communicate. Acknowledging and discussing the anger may dramatically relieve that block. Again, a statement such as "You appear to be angry today" may be all that is needed. If you know what at least some of the anger is about, it is helpful to say so. For example, patients who come to clinics at teaching hospitals frequently see students or residents they have not seen before. Patients might be angry about this, but usually won't say so unless permission is given. This is done with comments such as "It must be hard to see so many different doctors" or "It sounds as if you may be irritated that Dr. X is not here to see you again."

Emotions tend to provoke similar emotions in others. Fear is contagious. One responds to love with affection. Hostility and violence beget hostility and violence. An angry patient provokes anger in his or her doctor. A doctor may feel angry toward certain patients, but he or she should not express that anger. This will be discussed further in Rule 6.

5. *Feelings are usually acknowledged when that is suppportive to the patient.* A severely depressed patient reported that she had organized, cooked, and served an entire meal. The doctor responded to the report by saying "I can understand why you feel pleased about this." Since preparing meals is an ordinary task for some, it is easy to forget that this is a major new accomplishment for someone coming out of a depression. For a patient who has a demanding job, a statement such as "It is good that you could come today" can be supportive.

6. *The doctor rarely, and then only carefully and with much forethought, discloses his or her own feelings to the patient.* Doctors should

not tell patients they are angry unless they expect to accomplish something by this. It might be therapeutic for a patient to know that what he or she says and does makes others angry. If the patient is told this, it must be done in a nonpunitive way.

Occasionally, a patient will say ''I really want to know. How do you feel about me?'' Beware: this may be a trap. The patient has a preconceived idea of how the physician feels and this is what he or she expects to hear. Or, the patient may not really want to know. It is better not to respond directly to such a question, but instead to say ''Why do you ask?'' or ''What are your thoughts about that?'' As we have said before, the important facts are the patient's own thoughts and feelings. These determine how he or she behaves in the world.

7. *Occasionally a patient may need help in maintaining control of his or her emotions.* I usually encourage patients to express their feelings and it is of benefit for them to do so. Sometimes, it is better to do the opposite. That is, encourage the patient to exert more control and let the feelings out more slowly. A patient might feel guilty if too much hostility is expressed all at once toward the doctor. The same is true of amorous feelings. A patient who is encouraged to express all of his or her erotic feelings toward the doctor early in therapy might feel too guilty to return.

In most interviews, there is a melodic interplay among feelings and narrative. The best of these requires an aware patient and an aware interviewer. At the very least, the interviewer should not stop the patient from this interplay unless the patient may be getting out of control, and this is rare.

The doctor must, whether he or she wants to or not, cope with feelings that the patient brings and his or her own feelings engendered by the patient's attitudes and behavior. This is true no matter what specialty one practices. The following report by a medical student of his encounter with a patient in the medicine clinic illustrates how important it is for a student to be aware of his or her own feelings. The reader is free to judge how well everyone's feelings were handled in this encounter. The interview is taken verbatim from the student's write-up because it also expresses his own feelings so well.

It was mid-morning in the cardiac clinic and the waiting room was still crowded. I opened the door of room 315 and called for a Mrs. O. No answer. I checked the name on the chart and called again, several decibels louder. Still no answer. I called a third time and was about to despair when I saw the American Red Cross coming to my assistance. That is, the Red Cross nurse had approached an elderly, thin, gray-haired lady on the front row—only a short distance away—and with gestures and instructions voiced directly into the woman's hearing aid, was indicating to her that she had been called. Even after this was made clear to her, there seemed to be some additional reluctance to comply on the part of the patient. As the nurse delivered her to the door, the patient muttered something in a low voice which I could not hear clearly. But the nurse gasped and said, "Why you ought to be ashamed to say that!" and I was not formulating a paranoid delusion to suspect that the patient's comment had been less than complimentary regarding her first appraisal of me. This was soon verified. Instead of accepting my usual invitation to be seated on the bed, Mrs. O stood adamantly just inside the door and demanded, "Where is my doctor? You're not the one who saw me last time."

This series of opening maneuvers placed me on the defensive side of the scrimmage line, and my immediate reaction (feeling that it was necessary to do something) was to fumble through the chart as if in an effort to see just who this patient's healer was and to secure his services for her with all dispatch. However, even when I found the most recent clinic note, I could not recognize the signature from gross inspection, or even decipher it from close inspection, and was left to try to regain my composure and to say, "I'm sorry; he is not here today. I am assigned to examine you."

"You're not my doctor," she reasserted.

"I *am* your doctor for today, Mrs. O," I said more firmly, "and (without noting whether she was convinced of this or not) . . . how have you been getting along since we last saw you?"

Thus, my tedious hour with Mrs. O was underway, and with fluctuations to both sides of this baseline, a similar atmosphere prevailed throughout the interview. A 73-year-old white woman, the patient had the same complaints as when first seen in cardiac clinic five months previously: "soreness of the heart," and swelling of the feet and legs. The first words on her chart were, "The patient is a very poor historian," and this situation likewise seemed unchanged. In fragments extracted from a plethora of multiple aches and pains, it was ascertained that a nonangina-like, nonpleuritic, nondescript left anterior chest pain persisted ("The medicine is not doing any good") and that her legs were both still swollen—only the right one not so badly. Superficial inspection revealed obvious varicosities and a several centimeter difference in the leg circumferences. On further questioning, it was learned that the patient had had bilateral phlebectomies at another hospital six years ago and had not conveyed this information to the staff of this clinic. Regarding her surgeon at the other hospital, Mrs. O vehemently commented, "He sure made a mess of things, didn't he? The last time I saw him I told him to go to hell, and I always wondered if he did."

The physical examination was also accomplished with some difficulty. Mrs. O proved to be a sensitive creature who felt the lightest palpation as mortal pain, especially the percussion of the cardiac border over vulnerable left chest. I inquired into the nature of a small nodule over a posterior rib near the spine and Mrs. O promptly ordered me to direct my attention elsewhere, as this had been operated upon many years ago and "No doctor is going to cut on me again." During the presentation period the resident spent considerable time in trying to inspire me to hear a faint diastolic murmur in the primary aortic area. Mrs. O was exasperated because we seemed to be ignoring the true locus of her pathology and pointed out "It's not there; it's the left side that hurts," with "you stupid fools" implied in the tone of her voice.

Interjected several times into the latter portion of the examination was Mrs. O's demand that we hurry, for a neighbor had brought her to the clinic; the neighbor had to go to work at 2:00 PM; that she had been there all morning, etc. This made it doubly difficult when I allowed the patient to return to the waiting room and then had to call her back when the resident decided a blood sample should be drawn for a serum K + . To this proposal Mrs. O dogmatically stated that "They've got all of my blood reports already." This was the nth time that she had implied that I was essentially ignorant of her chart content and that much of the time had been wasted due to my lack of familiarity with her case. I took the opportunity for rebuttal and (not without a moment's contemplation) said half angrily, "Lady, don't you realize that what your blood showed one month ago has nothing to do with what it will show today and that this is done for your own benefit?"

Mrs. O was rather taken aback at the worm's turning and did not reply. The venipuncture was accomplished with a single shriek from the patient, and without further exchange the session was adjourned. On filling the blood chemistry tubes, I discovered that I had inadvertently used a 20cc instead of a 10cc syringe and had drawn twice as much blood as needed. It was inadvertent, but I wondered if some subconscious motivation had not been at work.

Feelings are always present and, in one way or another, will influence a doctor–patient encounter.

Nonverbal Communication

Part of the total gestalt and an important part of the interview is nonverbal information obtained by the physician as the patient is observed. Nonverbal behavior must be evaluated along with verbal information and within the context of the entire setting.

A number of books have been written about body language and facial expression. A quick review of them can alert you to various possibilities that you can then begin to observe and experience.

A cognitive knowledge of types of behavior is important, but not sufficient. The doctor–patient interaction is a total experience, part of which the doctor experiences and learns on a nonverbal level. One may understand the strokes of a tennis game by reading a description. This is helpful, but one only becomes adept at tennis by playing.

The beginning interviewer should pay special attention to whether or not nonverbal communication coincides with verbal communication. Discrepancies provide some of the best clues to what a person is feeling and may show feelings unknown to the patient.

"The most important aspect to all the systems is the notion that nonverbal behaviors convey information that, although in some cases redundant to spoken language, often provides additional information to that from verbal channels." (Harper et al 1978). Discrepancies between spoken words and nonverbal behavior tell the interviewer that what is said is not the entire story or may not be the story at all. In the initial interview, the patient may be wary of expressing his or her feelings. What he or she says may convey a general, but diluted statement of true feelings. Often, nonverbal behavior more nearly communicates deep feelings. Expressions of anger or sadness around the eyes are good things to look for.

The eyes are probably the most communicative area of the face. Eye contact is important. It is usually a signal that some contact is desired, that the patient is willing to communicate. Gaze avoidance may be a signal that the patient does not want to communicate. If gaze avoidance occurs toward the end of the interview, it may mean the patient wants to stop. In other words, looking encourages interaction and not looking discourages it. It can be a signal from patient to doctor or, at times, from doctor to patient.

Many authors have commented on the typical depressed attitude in the brows. The medial corners of the eyebrows are raised and drawn together sometimes creating an inverted "V" in the eyelid just below the brows. This may often be seen in patients who express no sadness or depression verbally. Although depression may be expressed only in the eyes, sometimes the mouth is drawn down and there may be trembling in the lower lip (Ekman and Friesen 1975). Other emotions are accompanied by characteristic facial expressions. We have a largely intuitive understanding of such expressions, but much can still be learned by studying the literature on the subject. According to Knapp, "The face is rich in communicative potential . . . next to human speech, it is the primary source of giving information. . ." (Harper et al 1978). Facial expression may be an innate characteristic of humans, cutting across cultures. In this way, it differs from other aspects of behavior which are culture-bound.

Charles Darwin's 1872 work, *The Expression of Emotion in Man and Animals*, put forth the theory that the facial expression of emotions is similar among species. More recent work has corroborated this idea. Darwin's was the first scientific approach to understanding facial expression in animals and man. The work, an instant "bestseller," was the culmination of years of painstaking observation. Here are some examples of what facial expressions tell us during an interview.

A woman tells of a terrible argument she had with her husband. As she starts talking, she is appropriately angry and a bit tearful. As she speaks more of her husband's anger and frustration, a slight smile creeps onto her lips:

DOCTOR: I guess John was pretty upset too.

PATIENT: Yes, he was, but I was mad because he didn't seem to appreciate how hard I worked. (Smile continues.)

DOCTOR: I know you were very upset, but maybe you also enjoyed getting back at him.

PATIENT: He thinks I don't do anything all day.

The last statement indirectly confirms the doctor's hypothesis derived from the patient's nonverbal behavior: that she enjoyed seeing her husband upset. She had retaliated indirectly for his perceived lack of understanding. This does not mean that the patient enjoyed the entire episode. Actually, she was very upset by it. Nevertheless, the satisfaction from seeing her husband angry was there. This vignette demonstrates that a bit of behavior may have several conflicting motives. The doctor does not necessarily systematically discuss all of these motives. It may be sufficient to allude indirectly to some of the conflicting motives, as demonstrated with this patient.

The following report of a medical student's interview with her patient is another example of how a patient may derive pleasure from adversity. An 81-year-old woman was seen in a medical clinic with mildly increased blood pressure and symptoms of hyperventilation syndrome. Because she was somewhat depressed and had great self-pity, the student had asked her to return the following week to the medicine clinic to discuss some of her problems. The material is presented verbatim from the student's written report of the interview:

> The patient had not been told that this interview was to be any different from any other medicine clinic visit. I had intended to slip naturally into our talk after taking a blood pressure. However, the patient began to talk immediately and no such subterfuge was ever necessary. Despite her numerous physical symptoms, she never seemed to miss the physical examination, and when she left I had the impression that she was relieved and pleased and had accomplished whatever she had come to do.

> STUDENT: How have you been since I saw you, Mrs. C?

> PATIENT: Not very good; I've been suffering terrible. My back hurts, (etc., etc.). I've been suffering terrible (etc.) (Each time the phrase was used, it was followed by a smile of modest martyrdom.)

> STUDENT: Didn't that medicine I gave you help any?

PATIENT: I didn't take it; it burned my throat.

STUDENT: How are things at home?

PATIENT: I have my own kitchen and bedroom that my son built for me, and I manage to be up and about. I do all of my own cooking and cleaning. I take care of myself. I don't work a hardship on nobody. (After a slight lull) Tell me doctor, does eating eggs cause arthritis to hurt?

STUDENT: I never heard of it.

PATIENT: I knew it! My son has been told by certain people that it did—she thinks she knows so much.

STUDENT: Who is she?

PATIENT: His wife. (Her look of triumph was obvious and I could sense her eagerness to get back into the fray with this new weapon.)

STUDENT: You and your daughter-in-law don't get along so well?

PATIENT: No; I try to, but she's awfully jealous.

Here is an example of how a patient's smile and "look of triumph" betrayed some of her real feelings about what she said was a difficult situation. We can be sure that the situation was difficult. It is not unusual to have mixed and even opposing feelings at the same time. No one likes to suffer, yet some people have learned that through their own suffering they can manipulate interpersonal situations to be pleasurable.

Experimental evidence confirms the validity of facial expression as an index to emotion. Schwartz, after placing electrodes on facial muscles, instructed subjects to think of sad, happy, or angry experiences. Even though no visual changes were detected in this experiment, physiologic readings of muscle reactions could differentiate among emotional states (Schwartz et al 1974).

Electromyographic recordings from skeletal muscles in all parts of the body have amply documented skeletal muscle response to emotion. As in the experiment by Schwartz, all muscle responses are not easily apparent, and the observer may not readily detect the facial expression of sadness or happiness. Instead, if you look carefully, you may see an overly controlled, somewhat rigid expression, something not infrequently seen in politicians. This, too, is an important piece of information: there is something else below the surface. Sometimes the simple question "What are your feelings about that?" will be enough to bring out these feelings.

Psychophysiological techniques have progressed beyond the mere documentation of physiological responses in emotion. Biofeedback can now help patients learn when they are anxious and tense and then learn to relax certain tense muscle groups by monitoring the electronic signals they produce. Patients with tension headaches have probably benefited from biofeedback therapy more than any other group.

Some psychologists, beginning with the James–Lange theory of emotions, have postulated that the physiological state precedes and is the basis of emotion. Facial movements and other neurological stimulation are presumed to set up proprioceptive responses that feed back to the central nervous system, stimulating the central feeling of emotion (James and Lange 1922). Using this theory, one would say that a facial configuration was the first expression of an emotional state, with the feeling tone being a later expression. I am not a proponent of this theory, but merely cite it to underline the importance of training oneself to study nonverbal behavior in order to understand better a patient's communications.

Although we tend to watch facial expressions more and get more information about a patient's emotions from them, other aspects of nonverbal behavior communicate important feelings. The interviewer should always observe the patient's walk and bearing when he or she enters the room. Walk can be the first clue the physician has of neurological and musculoskeletal disorders. It may also tell something about how the person relates to authority figures. The entire walk, bearing, associated movements, and facial expression certainly tells something about how the patient feels about the psychiatric interview and himself or herself in relation to it.

Personal space is an interesting aspect of nonverbal communication. Feelings about personal space probably relate to basic instincts of territoriality. The need for surrounding space varies with the relationship to individuals in the area, the culture, and feelings of the person. Psychiatric patients need more interpersonal space or they will tend to be more agitated. Paranoid patients require more social distance. Hall (1966) describes four distance zones. The intimate, close to 6–18 inches; personal distances, 1.5–4 feet; social distances, 4–12 feet; and public distances, 12–25 feet. These dimensions vary with culture. The French and Latin Americans have a much closer social distance. North Americans find themselves backing away from Latin Americans who come close for social conversation. Latin Americans may interpret this as coolness or hostile withdrawal.

Because psychiatric patients are more likely to interpret the behavior of others in terms of their own special emotional problems, an interviewer should be aware of any intrusions into their social and personal space. Conversely, it is important to note the patient's use of social and personal space. Fearful and paranoid patients are wary of coming too close. Other patients may want a closer encounter with their therapist than the situation calls for. This should alert the interviewer to the patient's need for love and protection or desire for an amorous relationship.

Personal space needs, body movement, facial expression, together with words are a panorama of behaviors to be evaluated. Sometimes all of them in concert may create a powerful effect on the interviewer. At other times, disparate behaviors signal a puzzling array of conflicts to be understood.

Relaxed Attentiveness

The meaning of the word "listening" may seem self-evident, but there are many ways to listen. The interviewer can listen for details and focus attention on specific areas. Or, he or she can hang on every word. Such focused attention tends to exclude information the patient might communicate because it narrows the areas of the interviewer's awareness. Specific focus is necessary from time to time in the interview, but if it is present all the time, it blocks observation of important relationships and discontinuities such as sequence of topics, the dropping of topics, what is not said, and congruences of nonverbal behavior. Attention to details should not exclude awareness of the doctor's own feelings and associations in response to what the patient says. Instead of constant focused attention, I recommend relaxed attentiveness. This is a kind of listening somewhat like the relaxed, but alert, attitude a person might have walking through the mountains. It takes in everything, but still allows the scene to develop and take on a meaning of its own. It also permits the doctor's own free associations to come into his or her awareness.

Part of the data a doctor works with when he or she interviews a patient is the free associations emanating from his or her own unconscious. Some might call this intuition. I call it clues from the doctor's random thoughts. Everyone should be permitted the freedom to experience these associations, to pay attention to them, to use them as clues, and then to look for further corroboration. These associations should never be considered true and correct statements. Dogma and prejudice lie in that direction. But, paying attention to them may lead the interview in interesting and fruitful directions and, at the same time, keep interviewers out of traps that occur when they are not aware that they may be projecting their own thoughts.

The schizophrenic patient who said he came in because he had blisters on his feet later said he thought he might be Jesus, but that he was different from Jesus because he had money in the bank and gold. Then, one by one, he began pulling gold rings from his pocket and placing them on the fingers of his right hand until there was a ring on each finger. What could be the meaning of this behavior? Was he trying to impress us with his wealth, and if so, why? We don't know, but our free associations are worth noting as clues as to what to listen for in the future. The associations of one member of the group went as follows: Christ was crucified. If the patient thinks he is Jesus, then he is in danger of being crucified, but he says he is different. He has gold rings, which he displays when he feels vulnerable. Certainly one would feel vulnerable when being interviewed by a group of medical students. Perhaps he feels quite vulnerable much of the time and uses the rings as a symbolic way of warding off threats.

What do you do with this type of conjecture? Use it conservatively—very conservatively. Remember, you may be wrong. First look for information to substantiate or refute the hypothesis. Then, when you feel you have data to substantiate what you are thinking, *do not tell the patient*. Your insights do him or her little good. They must be the patient's insights. Use your information as a guide to listening and to raise questions and stimulate patients to think about themselves in ways they may not have done before.

Relaxed attentiveness or free-floating attention, as it is sometimes called, also allows the interviewer to make tentative connections among what may at first seem to be unrelated material. I have already stated that interviewers know they are on the right track if their comments facilitate continuing discussion and further elaboration of what their patients had been talking about. As the patient talks, you need to pay attention not only to the content but also to the sequence of material—what material follows what. The patient's associations may very well be a clue to his or her motivations or they may help to explain some previously unexplained behavior.

A patient talks about how upset she is that she cannot seem to get a reaction out of her husband. She wants him to talk with her about the things that bother her about their relationship. She keeps trying to talk with him, but he doesn't seem to want to. Eventually, he gets angry with her and may yell or stomp out of the house. She says she doesn't understand why he doesn't want to talk with her. Next, she begins talking about how she was always getting into trouble as a child and she didn't realize she was doing something wrong until her mother yelled at her or spanked her and then she felt very angry. She felt she had been wronged and that her parents didn't understand. This sequence of content areas gives us a clue that wanting a reaction from her husband may, in some way, be related to the reactions she seemed to provoke in her parents. When she was "unjustly accused," she could feel righteously angry. If you treat these seemingly disconnected topics as if they were unrelated, you would miss a clue to some important psychodynamics.

Relaxed attentiveness also allows the interviewer to associate other elements in the sequence of the patient's discussion and consider possible connections. The interviewer might conclude that, for some reason, the patient did not want to discuss a topic just dropped. Do you try to get the patient to return to the first topic or allow him or her to continue on the changed subject? That's difficult to say. The first topic may be too painful to discuss, particularly in the early interviews. It is usually best to make a mental note and allow the patient to proceed. As the doctor–patient relationship grows you can say, "I notice you changed the subject. Any special reason?" Such defenses are never openly challenged if the patient continues to want to use them.

Other forms of communication commonly arise during an interview. If a patient constantly brings up a subject, even though the discussion has left that for a while, then the subject obviously has special meaning to the patient and you might inquire into this. A comment such as, "I notice you keep returning to that. Is there more you would like to say about it?" or "How might you like to solve that problem?" are possibilities. Inconsistencies are another area to be noted as the interview progresses, but, as I have said, you are not out to trip the patient up, nor should you confront patients directly with inconsistencies. Again, they are worth noting and bringing up at the appropriate time.

Relaxed attentiveness increases the likelihood of recognizing these and other aspects of the communication process.

Empathy and Sympathy

Empathy is the ability to put one's self in another's place and to view and feel about the situation as the other does. Empathy has a special quality about it. It is as if one *were* the other person for a brief moment. Sympathy is the sharing of the same feeling with another, but it does not involve the more global understanding and identification that empathy does. The doctor can use the understanding of empathy to help the patient to better understand his or her self and to learn to cope.

Sympathy may sometimes help the patient to feel better, but sympathy is more commiseration and does not imply help to move to a better adjustment. Sympathy may even discourage the patient from moving to a better adaptation by granting more legitimacy to the patient's feelings than is warranted. At other times, sympathy may actually discourage a patient from expressing feelings.

> Mrs. Edwards, a woman of 30, had had two successful pregnancies followed by two spontaneous abortions. She was pregnant for the fifth time when her father, who lived in the same house, died. Soon after this she threatened to abort. The doctor, who

had attended both father and daughter throughout, felt very sorry for her and put himself out to show his concern—among other ways, by bringing an obstetrician on a domiciliary consultation. The abortion, however, duly took place.

For the next two years the doctor saw no more of Mrs. Edwards. When she did return to him complaining of headaches, he saw from her records that she had chosen to consult his partners in the interval, attending with a variety of ill-defined symptoms. The doctor encouraged her to talk, and at length she burst out, "Don't waste your sympathy on me—I'm not worth it! I've wanted to tell you this for so long. My father was a very difficult man to live with and part of me was glad when he died. And I didn't want to hold on to that pregnancy either. But I felt so bad about it I couldn't possibly tell you when you were being so kind and sympathetic." (Freeling and Harris 1984, p 50)

In this case empathy, rather than sympathy, may have led to a better understanding of the woman's true feelings.

Empathy is essential to the doctor–patient relationship and to the progression of the interview. Showing empathy by comments, questions, and nonverbal behavior allows an interview to flow smoothly and unfold in a way that is beneficial to the patient. Failure to show empathy and to explore psychosocial information deprives the patient of the opportunity to share what that person feels about their illness with the doctor. Crouch and McCauley found that family-practice residents missed numerous opportunities to show empathy and to connect psychosocial information with health and illness. They cite the following example from a study of audiotaped interviews.

PATIENT: When I was 17 I had an ulcer and it started to bleed.

DOCTOR: How did they know you had an ulcer then?

PATIENT: Well, my Dad went to Vietnam . . .

DOCTOR: Uh-huh.

PATIENT: . . . and I guess that, uh, bothered me. When I was 15, uh, I was engaged to a guy that was in the military and he went to Vietnam. He was there for four months and he got killed.

DOCTOR: How did they know for sure it was an ulcer?

Neither the psychosomatic nor the psychosocial aspects of this topic were brought up again during the rest of the visit. (Crouch and McCauley 1986)

Poole and Sanson-Fisher (1979) state, "Acute empathy, genuineness and non-possessive warmth . . . are important aspects of interviewing and therapeutic process." Yet, students are not being trained in these.

In some medical schools students receive no training in this. This interferes with their ability to understand and treat the patient. As one patient said, "He [the student] seemed more interested in getting answers to his own questions than he was in trying to find out about my concerns and worries." Students can, however, be trained to have better empathy, and this leads to responses that are more appropriate to the patient. We might say that empathy is the lubricant that permits the doctor and patient to work well together and the interview to flow smoothly.

Taking Notes

Should students take notes, and, if notes are taken, how much information should they record and in what detail? Ideally, one would take no notes so that attention could be focused entirely on the patient. A study that rated videotaped interviews with and without note-taking "clearly indicates that sessions conducted without note-taking were seen by raters to be significantly higher on therapist effectiveness, client reaction to the session, and total therapeutic impact" (Hickling et al 1984).

Nevertheless, information obtained by the clinician must be recorded in order to be useful to the interviewer or to others treating the patient at a later date. A suggested outline for obtaining and recording psychiatric history data was given earlier. Other outlines using somewhat different forms of organization are available in psychiatric texts for comparison. Questions always arise as to how much to record and how to best retain the vast amount of information resulting from an interview. The history and mental status cannot be entered on the chart while one is interviewing the patient—at least not by medical students during their initial experiences with the doctor–patient relationship and the psychiatric examination. An experienced clinician who knows what to put down and what to leave out can sometimes do it, but the student is advised not to try.

Some interviewers have excellent recall and can therefore retain enough of the information from the interview to record what is necessary. Most, however, find it helpful to take a few notes during the interview. If done carefully, taking notes need not disrupt the interview. If the interviewer's complete attention and focus is on the patient, then he or she can jot down a few notes here and there to aid later recall without interrupting the patient's flow or interfering with his or her own attention to the patient's verbal and nonverbal cues. I do recommend one exception: a brief statement of the present illness should be recorded in the patient's own words and his or her own words should be used occasionally in other parts of the history.

Taking notes, however, should never become an end in itself. Some interviewers are so concerned with getting the material down on paper in the proper sequence and filling in all the blanks that they forget that patients are people who need to be encouraged to say what their problems are and what are on their minds in their own particular way and at their own speed. I once observed a doctor who, when the patient began talking about his feelings about some of his failures in life, quickly looked down his three quarters of a page of notes, spotted an incomplete place and said, "Now just a minute here, we still haven't found out what happened to you between the time you were last discharged from the hospital and when you moved to Florida." This doctor was too preoccupied with filling in the blanks and was unable to get anything but a few rather sterile facts from this patient. If you cannot allow a psychiatric patient to express feelings, you will not be able to help him or her, no matter how well a history is recorded on the medical chart.

Some interviewers will find that they cannot adequately concentrate on the patient if they are taking notes at all and that they work better with their patients without paper and pencil. In that case, if your recall is not adequate, a good compromise might be to take a few notes during the first interview or part of the first interview so that certain essential data is not lost, and then relinquish the note pad. If the interview is recorded immediately after the patient leaves, all material will not be lost.

PATIENTS' RESPONSE TO NOTE-TAKING

Most patients expect doctors to record a certain amount of information and, therefore, are not at all disturbed when their doctor takes notes. It often aids the relationship simply to say to the patient, "Would you mind if I take a few notes?" Most patients do not mind. This is a good time to explain to the patient that all of the material that comes from this interview will be confidential between the two of you, that you will not record on the chart anything that the patient does not want recorded, and, as a matter of fact, much of the material discussed will not be put down in the record.

Medical records are supposed to be confidential, but it seems that more and more they are becoming public information. Insurance companies feel that they must have a certain amount and kind of information before they will pay for medical treatment. Hospital records go through many hands. All those who have access to the records are supposed to maintain confidentiality. Mostly they do, but there is always the possibility of a breach in that confidentiality. In a teaching hospital where students, physicians, housestaff, and various technicians work with the patients and their records, you quickly learn that all medical information is not kept as confidential as you might like. For these reasons only the minimal necessary information for diagnosis and treatment of the patient should be put in the chart. Material about family and personal relationships should be alluded to only in general terms unless specific information about this is crucial for future therapy. Details on personal history, sexual life, and past transgressions are best left out, whenever possible.

Many psychiatrists keep their own personal record file apart from the official medical record. Every once in a while, as some of you may recall, these files figure in certain cloak and dagger scenarios. Files in any doctor's private office, of course, are not subject to the same possibility of being read by unauthorized persons as are those from an institution.

All patients should know what is recorded about them and who might have access to the material. Essentially, the people who have access to the material are medical personnel and, with the patient's permission, insurance companies and possibly others. Patients must give their permission for any information to be turned over to a third party and, even if the patient does give permission, it is the physician's responsibility to review carefully any information that is given and to be sure that it will not be harmful to the patient.

Some patients do not want anything recorded about them or they want to know specifically what is recorded. Their feelings should be taken into consideration. If they are not, the doctor–patient relationship cannot progress and it will be impossible for the patient to develop a therapeutic relationship. Some paranoid patients are afraid of how the recorded information will be used. In this case, carefully explain the purpose of the record to the patient and enlist his or her help in deciding what might be put into that record. Usually when this is done, the patient's concerns about the record disappear and what might be recorded is no longer an issue in the doctor–patient relationship.

Prominent and important people sometimes prefer that no records be kept of their psychiatric treatment; some of them will even go so far as to pay for their treatment in cash so that their name will not be on a bill from a psychiatrist. Certain corporations will jeopardize promotions or even fire an executive or employee who they find has had treatment for any mental problem. Public education should eventually be helpful in informing these groups, but, in the meantime, you must respect the patient's desire not to have his or her future with a company put in jeopardy.

References

Barsky AJ, Kazis LE, Freiden RB, Goroll AH, Hatem CJ, Lawrence RS: Evaluating the interview in primary care medicine. *Soc Sci Med* 1980;14A(6):653–658.

Binjs R, Sluijs EM, Verhaak PF: Byrne and Long: a classification for rating the interview style of doctors. *Soc Sci Med* 1984;19(7):683–690.

Carpenter WT Jr, Sacks MH, Strauss JS, Bartko JJ, Rayner J: Evaluating signs and symptoms: comparison of structured interview and clinical approaches. *Br J Psychiatry* 1976;128:397–403.

Cox A, Hopkinson K, Rutter M: Psychiatric interviewing techniques II. Naturalistic study: eliciting factual information. *Br J Psychiatry* 1981;138:283–291.

Crouch MA, McCauley J: Interviewing style and response to family information by family practice residents. *Fam Med* 1986;18(1):15–18.

Darwin CR: *The Expression of the Emotions in Man and Animals.* London, John Murray, 1872.

Ekman P, Friesen WV: *Unmasking the Face.* Englewood Cliffs, NJ, Prentice-Hall, 1975.

Freeling P, Harris CM: *The Doctor–Patient Relationship,* 3rd ed. Edinburgh, London, Melbourne, New York, Churchill Livingstone, 1984.

Haas AP, Henden H, Singer P: Psychodynamic and structured interviewing: issues of validity. *Compr Psychiatry* 1987;28:40–53.

Hall ET: *The Hidden Dimension.* Garden City, NY, Doubleday, 1966.

Harper RG, Wiens AN, Matarazzo JD: *Nonverbal Communication: The State of the Art.* New York, John Wiley & Sons, 1978.

Hickling LP, Hickling EJ, Sison GFP Jr, Radetsky S: The effect of note taking on a simulated clinical interview. *J Psychol* 1984;116(part 2):235–240.

James CG, Lange W: *The Emotions.* Baltimore, Williams & Wilkins, 1922.

Maguire GP, Rutter DR: History-taking for medical students I—Deficiencies in performance. *Lancet,* Sept 11, 1976, pp 556–558.

Poole AD, Sanson-Fisher RW: Understanding the patient: a neglected aspect of medical education. *Soc Sci Med* 1979;13A:37–43.

Schwartz GE, Fair PL, Greenberg PS, Mandel MR, Klerman GL: Facial expression and depression II: An electromyographic study. *Psychosom Med* 1974;37:81–82.

Sullivan HS: *The Psychiatric Interview,* Perry HS, Gawel ML (eds). New York, Norton, 1954.

5

Interviewing Across Cultural and Language Differences

Cervando Martinez, Jr., MD

Interviewing patients from different social, cultural, or language groups presents the interviewer with special challenges and opportunities. These include establishing rapport and adequate communication with someone different from oneself; comprehending a person's problems in the context of his or her sociocultural background; and providing the appropriate intervention without violation of sociocultural norms. The cross-cultural doctor–patient relationship, however, also provides the opportunity to learn about a person from a different group than one's own, to learn a modified set of interviewing skills, and to learn about the culture itself. The cross-cultural interview has the potential for a more rewarding outcome because of altered expectations and heightened interest, concentration, and awareness. And, as in all human interactions, certain pitfalls may lead to misunderstanding and a failure of communication.

The comments in this section are generally applicable to various groups: the poor, blacks, Hispanics, Asian Americans, and Native Americans, as well as more traditional members of other ethnic groups (i.e., Italian Americans). Because of my own experience, some emphasis will be placed on interviewing the Spanish-speaking patient.

As a general rule, the more like oneself a patient is, the easier it is to conduct an interview with that person. It is a human characteristic to feel affinity, rapport, and a sense of comprehension when encountering someone who shares something with us, whether it is having attended the same college, being from the same general social stratum, or having the same color skin. This is one reason why it feels good to meet a fellow countryman when traveling in a foreign country. This is a universal phenomenon and is not wrong. Most physicians and medical students in the United States come from middle-class backgrounds, speak English as their primary language, are white, and are obviously well-educated. However, the majority of people that medical students will have as patients during their years in training are from the lower class (medically indigent) and often are poorly educated. Blacks and other minority groups are overrepresented among the medically indigent. Thus, the interview across social-class, cultural, and language differences is important. However, a good interview is a good interview and the basic principles of patient interviewing and patient care apply to all groups. What this section contributes is an extra dimension, some special considerations, some information that may be useful, and a few specific techniques.

When conducting an interview with someone who is very much like oneself, the previously mentioned "instant rapport" occurs. "When the patient is from the same social class and ethnic group as the treating psychiatrist, therapy is often successful" (Foulks 1980). This sense of identification may be excessive (overidentification), however, and may produce difficulties. When a physician becomes ill, one of the difficulties involved in his or her care is this problem of too close an identification with the treating physician. The opposite often occurs when we interview someone who is very much unlike us. The sense of instant rapport and recognition is usually missing. Quite the opposite may be experienced by the interviewer: distant strangeness, awkwardness, puzzlement, or curiosity. A special effort must be made by both the doctor and the patient to bridge this distance. This brings us to the first basic principle of interviewing across sociocultural differences: the physician must first acknowledge to himself or herself that differences exist and that certain emotions may be present but are acceptable. The emotion felt during this sort of encounter may vary: a sense of general discomfort and unease, irritability, frustration, perhaps even anger.

Historically, most non-northern-European ethnic groups have had stereotypic characteristics attributed to them. These stereotypes may be complimentary (Asian Americans as industrious), but more commonly are pejorative (the cunning Japanese, the drunk Indian, the lazy Mexican). During the course of our socialization, each of us probably incorporates some of these notions without being fully aware of their presence. Physicians, being no different, may harbor them in some recess and should make every effort to be aware of these prejudices. What is harmful and must be guarded against is acting out these beliefs in the doctor–patient interaction. This can occur in many ways: by "accidental" slights, inattentiveness, carelessness, or even outright rejection and hostility. These and other damaging behaviors should be avoided.

What often may not be avoided, however, is the sense of puzzlement, unease, and the resulting frustration when dealing with a patient from a different social or cultural group. A useful technique in overcoming these feelings is to bring up the social and ethnic differences for discussion and explanation. The interviewer should not hesitate to say to a patient, ''I have not known very many people from your background and so we may have some difficulty understanding each other at first.'' This kind of statement acknowledges the differences between the doctor and the patient and the difficulties it may produce, but it also defines the problem as a joint one (''we may have some difficulty understanding each other'') and extends the possibility that it can be overcome (''at first''). It also opens the door for the patient to express his or her own concerns about being understood or misunderstood by someone so different. Indeed, the patient should be encouraged to express these concerns. (Patients may just as often have these same concerns about age differences.) This also sets the stage for the doctor to introduce the possible use of special techniques to improve communication: asking the patient to repeat or clarify certain things; asking the patient for specific information about culture habits and practice; or using an interpreter.

When working with any patient, the doctor should have some understanding of the patient's view (or explanation) of the condition producing his or her distress. Even highly educated persons are often uninformed or badly informed about health. People from other cultural groups may not only be poorly informed about medical matters, but may be operating with a conflicting explanation of disease. A common alternative explanatory model of disease is, of course, the religious/ supernatural: ''It is God's will that I am sick. I am being punished for my sins.'' A related perspective found among many Hispanics and some blacks involves the belief in the supernatural, witches, hexes, and evil spirits (*espiritismo*). The exact prevalence of these beliefs among various groups is difficult to judge accurately; however, the physician must know that these alternate models exist. They should be investigated to determine whether or not adherence to them interferes with proper medical management. Belief in folk illnesses, hexes, or other supernatural events, may coexist with belief in the scientific system and may not necessarily interfere with treatment. Likewise, many patients from certain cultural groups have faith in home remedies (amulets, poultices, herbs, teas, and the like). Most are harmless, but some may have significant therapeutic effects. Many of the herbs and teas used by Mexican Americans contain active naturally occurring substances. The therapeutic effect in most instances is determined by whether or not the individual has faith or believes in the remedy—an example of the placebo effect. Often the ritual, group and family involvement, catharsis, and support involved in a particular folk ritual may have powerful therapeutic psychological effects (e.g., the seances used by Puerto Rican *espiritistas*).

The use of interpreters when interviewing patients who do not speak English is controversial. Before an interpreter is used, determine if no communication at all can take place. For example, some non-English-speaking patients, when frightened, anxious, or in pain, attempt to protect themselves from these feelings by appearing helpless and less capable than they actually are of speaking English. A few words of the patient's language may serve to break the tension and demonstrate to the patient the interviewer's sincere interest in communicating. Pronouncing a patient's name correctly is also of great value. One's name is central to a sense of identity and self. If the English-speaking doctor correctly pronounces the patient's name, a great deal is said about the physician's respect for the patient's worth and dignity.

The form of address is also important. Mainstream American culture in the 1960s and 1970s changed dramatically in many ways, one of which was a relaxation of codes of social behavior. Relationships have become more casual and informal. Calling elders or superiors by their first name became more acceptable. This change in manners has not occurred among some cultural groups. It is still advisable when addressing an older patient to use the last name preceded by Mr., Mrs., or Miss. The Spanish language has formal and informal forms for verbs, nouns, and pronouns. Thus, there is a built-in emphasis on formality in human behavior. This adherence to more traditional forms of behavior carries over into personal relationships and has implications for the interview.

Interviewing the Family

In the social and cultural groups under consideration, particularly in their more traditional members, the family beyond the nuclear family is extremely important. Patients from these more traditional families come to us still enmeshed, in positive and negative ways, with parents, grandparents, in-laws, other relatives, and even godparents. There are special and powerful cultural norms guiding their family-oriented behavior, as in the emphasis placed on respect for elders in Japanese Americans. Furthermore, members of poor minority families, out of economic necessity, may be thrust into dependent relationships with family members that can result in considerable conflict, and if the economic aspects are ameliorated, significant pathology may not remain. It is thus a cliché to say that in the evaluation and treatment of the minority patient the family should be seen and worked with. This is fine and presents the usual problems if patient and family are willing to talk to the doctor. However, often, especially during an initial psychiatric evaluation the patient may not so readily agree to family involvement, and this then leads to a delicate clinical situation that, if not handled sensitively, may lead to difficulties in future care.

Most commonly encountered is the adult patient accompanied by a spouse or parent who expects either to enter the examination room or be privy to part if not all of the evaluation process. In other words, for whatever reason, personal, cultural, or some of both, the accompanying family member *expects* to be involved in what is going on without apparent regard to the question of doctor–patient confidentiality. Sometimes the patient appears grossly confused, mute, or uncooperative, and the physician may make the immediate decision to ask the entire family into the exam room for at least the initial part of the interview. Even in these cases, if the patient seems unwilling to have the family present it is best to start without them. At the other extreme are those cases where it seems advisable to interview the patient with the family present and the patient has no objections. If this occurs, it is still a good idea to ask the family to excuse themselves sometime during the interview to permit the patient the opportunity to be with the doctor in a freer climate. In all other cases (that is, when the patient's clinical condition does not appear to call for family presence initially) the patient is seen and then there arises the question of speaking to the family. This may be particularly troublesome when the patient does not want the doctor to speak to the family. This situation will not be dealt with here. Most commonly though, the patient has no strong objection and the family very much wants to play some part. The patient can be asked to specify any aspects of what has already been discussed that are not to be discussed with the family, and the physician may tell the patient that he or she wishes out of courtesy to talk to the family and invites the patient to be present. He or she may add that what the patient has disclosed will not be revealed but that the family's point of view may be useful.

Most families want to report what they have seen of the patient's behavior (especially in a psychotic process) that to them has been confusing and frightening. They wish an opportunity to receive some medical feedback and answers to basic questions. What is going on? Is the patient going to be all right? What can be done? What can they do to help? What does the doctor think the problem is?

Thus most families, particularly traditional ones, expect to see the physician and hear something about their relative's condition. The physician must take care not to needlessly retreat too far behind the curtain of confidentiality, thus losing the family and patient in the process. Finally, on interviewing the family, it is important to quickly determine who the most senior person appears to be and initiate the interview there even though this person may not necessarily be the most knowledgeable. Typically, this is the father, but the mother may really know more about what is happening. However, the father's position should be respected and addressed accordingly.

Diagnostic Considerations

Certain additional aspects of the content and process of the cross-cultural interview and the resulting data need to be delineated. Foremost is the effect of language differences on the information being gathered and the resulting influences on the diagnostic process. The diagnostic process is central to the delivery of medical care. Blacks and other large minority groups (Hispanics, Asian Americans, and Native Americans) have been overrepresented among the poor. The poor generally have a lower educational level than the national average of more than twelve grades. The disparities in educational level between poor patients and their physicians may create a gulf of misunderstanding. This can be a critical problem as medical care becomes more complex. This will become evident to the student as he or she tries to explain a drug regimen, the indications for cardiac surgery, or genetic risk factors to a patient with a fifth-grade education who is also distracted by the many hassles of being poor (long waits, public transportation, poor housing).

Eliciting complex symptom patterns from the patient during the history and review of systems enables the physician to rule out a large number of possible disease processes. The proper analysis of these symptom complexes as described by the patient in his or her own words involves the physician's mental processing of these perceptions into medical and scientific terms. This reprocessing is a form of translation that occurs all the time, but in the cross-cultural situation it may be more difficult. The analysis of information gathered by a physician from a black recruit, an elderly woman from China, or a Mexican worker in Texas involves several levels of reprocessing. Poor people and many members of minority groups speak a different form of English, if they speak English at all. It therefore behooves the physician to learn some of these variations of English and their medical application.

In general medicine, diagnosis involves synthesizing data from the history and review of symptoms with the signs found in the physical examination and laboratory data obtained later. In psychiatry, diagnosis is based on the reported symptoms, history, and so on, combined with the observations made in the mental status examination. Unlike data from physical examination and laboratory procedures, that obtained from the mental status examination remains largely verbal rather than observable physical changes and technical measurements. Thus, language continues to play a confounding role in psychiatry, and especially in the cross-cultural psychiatric interview and mental status examination.

The literature notes that poor and minority patients have a greater tendency to use somatization to deal with anxiety and to present with the somatic manifestations of anxiety, particularly tensionlike head and neck pain. This finding has been reported in several independent field studies of symptom patterns, and its reasons have not been completely explained. They may be an artifact. If not, they may be explained as a manifestation of a lower level of sophistication in verbal communication. Upper class (and better educated) minority patients do not demonstrate this tendency. There have been few other consistently demonstrated cross-cultural differences in symptom patterns among groups in the United States.

Other factors need to be kept in mind when performing the mental status examination and analyzing the data obtained. The assessment of appearance and general behavior during the interview can pose problems because a patient from a different social and cultural group will look and act differently from the examiner. The examiner must take into account his or her own ethnocentrism in evaluating whether a given observed behavior (clothing, hygiene, attitude, mannerisms) deviates from the norm for the patient's sociocultural group. This is similar to the sort of mental adjustments we make when assessing patients of different ages. There is socioculturally specific behavior just as there is age-specific behavior.

When examining a poor Appalachian patient, illiteracy, a shabby appearance, and a resigned attitude should not be interpreted as mental retardation, lack of concern for the self, or apathy. Wariness and irritability in a young black man are not paranoia and increased aggression. Some minority patients will become excessively passive and compliant when facing a stressful clinical situation that may remind them of a hostile or discriminatory environment they may have encountered. The line between psychopathology and socioculturally appropriate behavior is fine and variable. This is not to say that the majority of observations made during the cross-cultural interview are invalid; they are not. Pathology is pathology. However, some findings are more susceptible to distortion by language and social factors.

Demonstration of affect is one of these. Accurately and clearly translating feelings into words is very difficult for many patients, regardless of background. Add to this possible language differences and frequent lack of verbal sophistication and the result is the potential for distortion, blunting, or inappropriate expression. Some groups (e.g., traditional Japanese) emphasize a reserved demeanor. Others are more expressive (e.g., Cubans). Generally speaking, however, an interview conducted in the patient's preferred language will elicit a fuller, more intense, and clearer affective picture, and may demonstrate more or less pathology, depending on the situation. A predominantly English-speaking patient from a different social class than the examiner may likewise appear more constricted because of anxiety or guardedness based on class differences.

Assessment of thinking cross-culturally also presents some pitfalls. The patient who speaks another language or dialect of English may be translating simultaneously into English during an interview. This will tend to produce hesitations, vagueness, concreteness, disjointedness, or derailments. These findings may be interpreted as evidence of a thought disorder. Concreteness of thinking should be interpreted cautiously when observed in a cross-cultural interview because it may simply be a manifestation of literal translation, or lack of education, or both. Patients who do not speak or understand standard English well, often do poorly on the "formal testing" part of the mental status examination because of poor or inaccurate comprehension of test instructions. Finally, the assessment of intellectual level is fraught with problems because it is so dependent on verbal skills and vocabulary. A "social functioning" IQ assessment or testing by a bilingual examiner may provide a more accurate guide to intelligence.

Some psychiatric symptoms such as depersonalization or derealization and some delusions require a certain level of verbal ability for comprehensible expression. Therefore, patients who do not communicate well in standard English may have difficulty describing these symptoms to the examiner, and they might be considered less symptomatic. Cultural elements also get included in psychotic productions (e.g., delusions about laser beams, witches, and the like), but belief in the supernatural does not always mean psychosis.

The conclusion of an interview is as important as the beginning. It presents one last time where communication can break down. Then, however, it is communication from doctor to patient involving instructions, explanations, and directions. However, as I have tried to indicate, this potential for problems should also be seen as a clinical challenge and a stimulus for adapting our techniques to the patient's specific needs.

Reference

Foulks EF: The concept of culture in psychiatric residence education. *Am J Psychiatry* 1980;137:811–816.

Suggested Readings

Comas-Diaz L (ed): *Clinical Issues in Cross-Cultural Mental Health*. New York, John Wiley & Sons, in press.

Gaw A (ed): *Cross-Cultural Psychiatry*. Littleton, MA, John Wright, 1982.

Marcos LR, Urcuyo L, Kesselman M, Alpert M: The language barrier in evaluating Spanish-American patients. *Arch Gen Psychiatry* 1973;29:655–659.

Wilkinson CB (ed): *Ethnic Psychiatry*. New York, Plenum, 1986.

6

AMSIT: A Description of the Patient's Current Mental Status
David S. Fuller, MD

Overview

The mental status report or AMSIT (see outline) is a systematic documentation of the patient's thinking, feelings, and behavior at the time of the interview. These findings are particularly helpful to the clinician in deciding if a patient has evidence of mental retardation, an organic mental disorder, a psychosis, or a mood disorder. In addition, the description of such variables as how the patient relates to the examiner and the content of the patient's thinking help the reader to understand the patient's psychodynamics. Thus the report is of practical value not only in making a diagnosis but also in planning appropriate therapy.

As a description of current clinical findings, the AMSIT portion of a complete psychiatric case report is analogous to the description of physical examination findings. It is not a report of history. It also stands apart from conclusions concerning diagnosis and treatment.

The AMSIT organizes clinical findings into a systematic report that is written after the interview is completed; it in no way suggests the sequence of topics in the interview. A nondirective interview, for example, follows a course dictated by how the patient chooses to tell about himself or herself, and his or her problems and life experiences. The AMSIT outline, however, does provide the clinician with a checklist of mental functions to be evaluated before the interview's conclusion. While talking with the patient, the interviewer can thus be sure of having an observational basis of evaluating the patient's mood and affect, sensorium, current intellectual function, and several aspects of the patient's thought. If the patient's spontaneous comments fail to give the clinician an adequate basis for a conclusion about orientation, memory, fund of information, and abstracting ability, for example, specific questions should be asked to test these functions after the earlier, less-directive portion of the interview has been completed.

The AMSIT is written as five paragraphs, each under a major heading. Subheadings are not used.

OBSERVATIONS AND CONCLUSIONS

The AMSIT report contains both observations and conclusions based on inference. To say that the patient looked at the floor throughout the interview and never made eye contact with the examiner is to state a factual observation. On the other hand, to say that the patient is moderately depressed is to state a conclusion based on inference. Such a conclusion might, for instance, be inferred from observations such as the patient's dejected facies, lack of spontaneity, and by his statements about feeling sad and hopeless. *Conclusions and inferences should be substantiated with specific observations* whenever possible.

PRESENT TENSE

AMSIT findings should be described in the present tense. It is as though the one who writes an AMSIT is saying to the reader, "The patient is thinking, feeling, and behaving this way at this time."

PERTINENT POSITIVE AND NEGATIVE FINDINGS

Although it is not necessary to make a statement in the report about every possible observation, some description for each of the five major headings is always indicated. In addition, pertinent negative findings should always be recorded that help the clinician to rule in or to rule out the diagnostic possibilities that must be considered for the specific patient who is being described. For example, if the patient has clinical findings that suggest the diagnostic possibilities of bipolar disorder, manic type, and schizophrenia, the AMSIT should specifically state whether the patient does or does not demonstrate increased psychomotor activity, distractibility, clang speech, infectious elation, and flight of ideas (which are characteristic of mania) as well as whether the patient demonstrates neologisms, echolalia, blocking, loose associations, and impaired abstracting ability (which suggest schizophrenia).

AMSIT Outline

General Appearance, Behavior, and Speech

> *Appearance and behavior:* apparent age, sex, and other identifying features; appearance of being physically ill or in distress; a careful description of the patient's dress and behavior

Manner of relating to examiner: collaborative, placating, negativistic, distrusting, seductive, motivation to work with examiner

Psychomotor activity: increased or decreased

Behavioral evidence of emotion: tremulousness, perspiration, crying, clinched fist, turned-down mouth, wrinkled brow, and the like

Repetitious activities: mannerisms, gestures, stereotypy, cerea flexibilitas, compulsive performance of repetitious acts

Disturbance of attention: distractibility, self-absorption

Speech: easily understood, spontaneous, low volume, mutism, word salad, perseveration, echolalia, clang, affectation, neologisms

Mood and Affect

Mood

Position on the 7-point depression–elation continuum

Angry, fearful, or anxious mood

Affect: range, intensity, lability, appropriateness to immediate thought

Sensorium

Orientation: for time and place

Memory: for recent events especially

Serial 7 subtractions

(valid only if patient is adequately educated)

(also tests attention, intelligence, motivation)

Intellectual Function

Estimate current level of function as *above average, average,* or *below average* based on general fund of information, vocabulary, and complexity of concepts

Thought

Coherence

Logic

Goal directedness: tangential thought, circumstantiality

Associations: loose, pressured, or slowed thought, flight of ideas, blocking

Perceptions: hallucinations, ideas of reference, illusions, depersonalization, distortion of body image

Delusions

Content, other: major themes verbalized by the patient

Judgment

Abstracting ability: similarities, proverbs (be aware of limitations)

Insight: into the fact that the patient has a mental or emotional problem and into its nature

The Five AMSIT Sections

GENERAL APPEARANCE, BEHAVIOR, AND SPEECH

In the paragraph under this heading the clinician describes observations relative to these three general variables. A verbal picture should be painted that permits the reader to get a sufficiently clear image of the patient that the latter could easily be identified from a group of patients; for example, "This emaciated, elderly woman with uncombed grey hair, dressed only in a hospital gown, sits motionless in her chair, staring vacantly at the floor." A *description of how the patient relates to the examiner* should always be included. Valuable information is conveyed if the description of a patient's manner of relating includes some specifics; for example, it is informative to report that "The patient eagerly participates in the interview, relating to the examiner in an ingratiating, compliant manner." On the other hand, "The patient is cooperative," is so general as to give the reader little information. Describe any *increased psychomotor activity* (such as that seen in mania, in excited catatonia, and in some organic mental disorders) or *decreased psychomotor activity* (seen in "catatonic stupor," in some depressions, and in some organic mental disorders). The patient's psychomotor behavior should be described as increased or decreased only when there is a fairly gross deviation from the usual range of behavior.

Although another section of the AMSIT deals with mood and affect, *behavioral evidence of emotion* should be described here. For instance, anxiety may be suggested by recurrent laughter or by pupillary dilitation, hyperventilation, or chain smoking. Other examples of behavioral evidence of emotion appear in the outline.

Describe any unusual mannerisms or gestures demonstrated by the patient. *Stereotypy* (persistent mechanical repetition of speech or motor activity), *cerea flexibilitas* (waxy flexibility, in which limbs remain for a while in the position in which they are placed), and *compulsively repeated acts* should be described if present. Attention disorders include *distractibility*, in which attention is diverted in response to minimal provocation (seen in mania, anxiety states, and schizophrenia), and *self-absorption*, in which the patient is engrossed in himself to the point of inattention to other issues.

Disorders of speech include *decreased spontaneity, mutism* (refusal to speak), *word salad* (an incomprehensible mixture of words and phrases), *perseveration* (repetition of a verbal response to varied stimuli), *echolalia* (parrotlike repetition of the examiner's words), *clang* (words or phrases connected by the similarity of their sounds), *affectation* (artificiality of speech), and *neologism* (newly coined words created by the patient, often from parts of real words). It is appropriate to describe anything notable about the volume and pitch of the patient's voice and whether the patient's speech is clearly understood.

MOOD AND AFFECT

Mood refers to a *sustained* emotion. For practical purposes, the dominant emotion for the duration of the interview may be considered the patient's mood. First a statement should be made concerning which of the following seven possibilities best describes the patient's current mood:

> Severely depressed
>
> Moderately depressed
>
> Mildly depressed
>
> Euthymic
>
> Mildly elated
>
> Moderately elated
>
> Severely elated

The observational basis for any of the possibilities other than euthymic mood must be described. Any additional *sustained* emotion such as angry mood, fearful mood, or anxious mood should also be described.

Affect refers to an immediately expressed and observed emotion. Normally affect changes repeatedly through an interview, always in syncrony with what the person is currently thinking. For instance, a patient with no disorder of affect might feel sad when talking about the recent death of a loved one, then, a few minutes later, feel enthusiastic about a new job opportunity. Deviation from this normal pattern of moderately fluctuating but content-appropriate affect is highly significant in the psychiatric evaluation. The following four affect variables should always be described:

1. *Range of affect* refers to the extent to which both emotional highs (happiness) and lows (sadness or soberness) appear in the interview. A person with a decreased or constricted range of affect shows little emotional variation through the interview. The patient's range of affect is usually described as increased, decreased, or as neither increased nor decreased.

2. *Intensity of affect* can be thought of as the amplitude of emotional

expression. When a patient's feelings of sadness, anger, fear, anxiety, joy, and so on, are communicated with greater than usual amplitude, this is described as increased intensity of affect. Intensity may also be decreased or neither increased nor decreased.*

3. *Lability of affect* is evidenced by a rapid, extreme, brief change of emotion followed by a quick return to the previous level. A patient who, for example, has abrupt onset of crying followed by abrupt cessation of crying can be described as having a labile affect. Lability of affect is always an abnormal finding. A short burst of laughter when a patient is anxious is usually not an example of labile affect. In the AMSIT report a statement should be made indicating whether the patient does or does not have a labile affect.

4. *Appropriateness of affect* refers to whether the emotion at a particular moment is the one expected for the patient's currently expressed thought. For clarity, it is suggested that the statement concerning this variable indicate whether the patient's affect is or is not appropriate to the patient's thought at all points during the interview.

SENSORIUM

In this paragraph is described the examiner's evaluation of the patient's *orientation*, *memory*, and *calculating ability*. Impairment of one or more of these functions is described as impaired sensorium and suggests delirium or dementia. A statement should be included that indicates whether the patient's sensorium is clear or impaired.

If the patient's spontaneous comments fail to demonstrate conclusively that orientation and memory are intact, these functions should be tested. The patient should be able to state accurately and fairly quickly the correct month, date, and year. Missing the date by a day or so, or naming the previous month on the first of a new month is usually insignificant. The patient should also be able to state his current location. Although memory functions include immediate recall, recent memory, and remote memory, particular attention should be given to whether a patient can commit new items to memory and can recall them a few minutes to a few days later. Recent memory is a function that is almost always impaired in delirium and dementia. (Of course,

---

* Although the term *blunted affect* is sometimes used to describe moderately decreased range and intensity, and the term *flat affect* is used to describe markedly decreased range and intensity, it is suggested that range and intensity of affect be described individually because they are best thought of as independent variables.

memory may appear to be impaired in an unmotivated depressed patient, when, in fact, memory is unimpaired and sensorium is clear.) Recent memory can be tested by giving the patient five unrelated objects to remember that are not in the examining room. First the examiner asks for an immediate recall of the objects to make sure that the patient correctly understands them. Ten to fifteen minutes later, the examiner asks the patient to name the objects again. Memory can also be tested by asking the patient to recall the name of the examiner, to state the duration of his hospital stay, or to report other recently acquired information. When digit span is used to test recall, random numbers should be given at a rate no faster than one numeral per second. A normal person is expected to recall at least five digits forward and four backward.

Testing a patient's calculating ability (if the patient previously had the skill) is particularly useful in testing the sensorium. Because subtracting serially the number seven is most challenging, the patient is asked to subtract seven from 100, seven from the answer, and so on, repeatedly until six or eight subtractions have been completed. Although this tests concentration and intellectual ability also, it sometimes identifies early or mild organicity before the patient is disoriented for time and/or place.

Evidence of any other impairment of cognitive functions that suggests mental organicity should also be described in the Sensorium section if observed or elicited by testing.

INTELLECTUAL FUNCTION

The clinician evaluates the patient's current level of intellectual function on the assumption that below-average ability, regardless of its cause, impairs the patient from coping most effectively with the complexities of living. Although allowance is not made in the mental status evaluation for early-life brain damage, limited schooling, or lack of intellectual stimulation in childhood, these factors are considered in the global assessment at the end of the complete case report.

Intellectual function should be estimated, based on the patient's knowledge of *general information*, an observation of the patient's *vocabulary*, and on the extent to which the patient spontaneously *employs complex concepts*. The clinician should state whether the patient is judged to be functioning at the time of the interview in the average range (IQ approximately 85 to 115), above average (IQ greater than 115), or below average (IQ less than 85). The patient's spontaneous comments may demonstrate a substantial fund of information and thus make it unnecessary, or even inappropriate, to ask informational questions. To test the patient's general fund of information, the examiner may ask such questions as the following:

1. Name the president and vice president of the United States.
2. How many U.S. senators are there?
3. How many stripes are in the U.S. flag?
4. Name four of the largest cities in the United States.
5. What metal is attracted to a magnet?
6. What time of day is your shadow shortest?

The examiner may choose to ask other informational questions, particularly those that are consistent with the patient's experiences.

THOUGHT

This section is of particular importance in recognizing the presence of a psychosis, since psychotic patients have characteristic disturbances of thought. In addition, every patient's content of thought is noteworthy. The clinician should state whether the patient's thinking is *coherent*, *logical*, and *goal-directed*. Describe the patient's pattern of *associations*, and state whether there is evidence of *perceptual distortions* and/or *delusions* observed during the interview. In addition, describe the patient's other *content of thought*, *judgment*, *abstracting ability*, and *insight*. In order to be sure that each of these ten variables is described, it is suggested that the indicated sequence be followed as a matter of habit.

The first four variables involve the *form* of one's thinking, that is, how a patient's thoughts are organized and expressed. *Coherence* concerns whether one's thoughts stick together well enough that they easily make sense. *Logic* concerns whether one's conclusions are based on sound reasoning. It is, for instance, illogical to employ dichotymous, black-or-white thinking inappropriately. *Goal-directedness* concerns one's ability to pursue a definite goal in a direct fashion in the verbal expression of thought. With *tangential thought* the patient abandons his ideational objective in pursuit of thoughts peripheral to the original goal. With *circumstantial thought* the patient makes considerable detours with extraneous details but eventually reaches his thinking goal. Thought may be *pressured* (rapid) or *slowed*. Disordered patterns of associations include *flight of ideas* in which the patient rapidly jumps from one thought to another yet the thoughts are clearly connected (seen especially in mania), *loose associations* in which the examiner can discern little or no connection between ideas in the sequence (seen especially in schizophrenia), and *blocking*, which involves a sudden stop in the train of thought, often in mid-sentence.

Content of thought is of considerable importance in clarifying how the patient perceives his world, the nature of his conflicts, and how he is attempting to adapt. False perceptions include *hallucinations* (auditory, visual, or other sensory experiences in the absence of an external stimulus), *ideas of reference* (false beliefs that public events or messages refer to the patient), *illusions* (misinterpretations of sensory stimuli), *depersonalization* (feelings of unreality or strangeness concerning one's self), and *distortion of body image* (an erroneous internal picture of one's body or its parts). One should record here only those hallucinations, ideas of reference, and so on, that are experienced during the interview. *Delusions* are false beliefs that include ideas of persecution, grandiosity, poverty, and guilt. Again, only delusions held at the time of the interview are to be recorded here. In describing the patient's *other content of thought*, about four to six central themes should be listed, preferably in one sentence. Include both spontaneous and elicited thought content. Although the purpose is to describe the patient's thinking content at the time of the interview, this may sometimes include the patient's preoccupation with past events (for example, hallucinations that were experienced in the past). This is not, however, the place to describe the history of the present illness or the past history. For any depressed patient, a statement concerning the presence or absence of suicidal thinking during the interview should always be described with the content of thought.

Judgment involves the ability to make appropriate decisions concerning what to do in occupational, economic, and interpersonal situations. As an example, the patient could be asked, "What would you do if a lost three-year-old child appeared at the front door of your home?" The best tests of judgment are customized to the patient's life experiences. A housewife, for instance, might be asked how she would spend $40 to buy groceries for her family of six to last a week if there were no food in the house. *Abstracting ability* is the ability to think in generalizations. This is sometimes tested by asking the meaning of *proverbs* (to see if the patient gives an abstract rather than a concrete explanation). Because some cultural groups use proverbs uncommonly, a generally more valid method of testing abstracting ability involves asking the patient to identify the way in which objects are similar, for example, an apple and an orange or a table and a chair. The inability to think abstractly suggests the possibility of mental retardation, organic mental disorder, or schizophrenia. *Insight* is a correct understanding by the patient of the nature, cause, and extent of any mental or emotional problem that he or she may have. It is appropriate to indicate what the patient does and does not understand about his or her condition when describing his level of insight.

Sample AMSIT Reports
PATIENT 1

General Appearance, Behavior, and Speech

MW, an energetic and moderately obese 34-year-old white woman, makes a dramatic entrance wearing a wide-brimmed hat and a colorful Hawaiian muumuu. She carries a suitcase in one hand and a can of cola in the other. Before sitting, she greets each person in the room personally, making approving or critical remarks to each. Her rapid, voluble speech is punctuated by rhyming, puns, and clang. The patient looks directly at the examiner a great deal, pointing her finger for emphasis as she speaks. In addition to having an increased level of psychomotor activity, she is highly distractible. Twice she arises from her seat to examine and to comment on objects in the room. Occasionally she expresses intense anger. At one point, she remarks to the examiner, "Sonny, send for some coffee; I'll pay you well." Upon leaving, she pointedly shakes each person's hand and gives a personal message. She asks one student doctor if he would be against "messing around" with an older woman.

Mood and Affect

The patient's mood is severely elated with an infectious quality to it. Her elation is evidenced by vivacious movements, by the euphoria elicited in those with her, and by her content of thought (*q.v.*). The patient's affect is characterized by both increased range and intensity. Lability of affect is observed on two occasions when the patient demonstrates transient, deep feelings of sadness. Her affect is consistently appropriate to her thought content.

Sensorium

Ms. W's sensorium is clear as indicated by her correct orientation for time and place and by her excellent memory for recent events. Her ability to do serial seven subtractions is not tested.

Intellectual Function

The patient currently has above-average intellectual function as indicated by vocabulary (she uses "ostensibly" and "despoil"), complexity of concepts (she refers to multiple motives for a single bit of behavior), and fund of information (she mentions the three branches of the federal government).

Thought

The patient's thinking is coherent and generally logical, but it is never directed toward any single goal for more than about a minute. Her associations move quite rapidly from one subject to another in a manner that can be easily followed. She thus demonstrates true flight of ideas. She evidences no perceptual distortion such as hallucinations. Delusional thinking is indicated by her report of (*a*) her plan to sell dessicated long-stem roses that can be reconstituted, (*b*) a book she is writing about her life from which she expects to receive $500,000 in royalties, and (*c*) her recent telegram to the president announcing that she will drop by the White House next Monday to share her ideas for resolution of our country's problems in the field of foreign affairs. Other thought content includes her satisfaction with only three hours sleep per night, her colorful sexual experiences, her father's episodic psychoses, her "friendships" with famous people, and her recent consumption of five to six highballs daily. She tells several off-color jokes. Clearly impaired judgment is evidenced by her use of innapropriate behavior in the interview situation. Ms. W has good abstracting ability as demonstrated by her performance on both similarities and proverb interpretation. Her poor insight is indicated by her puzzlement as to why anyone would think that she needs to be hospitalized on a psychiatric unit.

PATIENT 2

General Appearance, Behavior, and Speech

Mr. E, an unkempt Chinese American man appearing to be his stated age of 20 years, is brought to the examining room only after 10 minutes of persuasion by the nurse. He wears a dirty tee shirt, blue jeans that are too large for his small frame, and sneakers without socks. He has about a four-day growth of beard, and his uncombed hair looks dirty. His facies suggest bewilderment and also distrust of the examiner. Only rarely does Mr. E look at the examiner. He generally speaks haltingly, but at times he negativistically refuses to speak while looking out the window. The patient speaks in a monotone with low volume. The examiner never gets the feeling that effective communication is established between them. Throughout the interview the patient repeatedly grasps his nose between his thumb and forefinger when speaking of himself. Agitation is evidenced by continuous hand movement and by the patient's walking about the room for brief periods while the examiner remains seated.

Mood and Affect

The patient's mood is mildly depressed as evidenced by his facies and by the feeling he elicits in the examiner. Affect is characterized by markedly decreased range and intensity. Although his affect is never labile, the patient shows almost no emotion when talking about issues that would be expected to be a source of strong feelings. At one point,

Mr. E demonstrates inappropriate affect by laughing at length while telling of having been committed to the state hospital.

Sensorium

After initially answering, "I don't know" to questions about the date, the patient gives the correct month, date, year, and name of this hospital. He correctly recalls the date he was admitted to the hospital, the name of his primary physician, and other details of the recent past. He recalls five digits forward and four digits backward. His sensorium is not impaired.

Intellectual Function

The patient's fund of information, concept formation, and vocabulary suggest he is currently functioning at an average intellectual level.

Thought

The patient's thinking is often incoherent, illogical, and without a clear direction in goal. His associations are also frequently loose. He uses newly coined words that have special meaning to him. Twice the patient asks the examiner to stop speaking so that he can hear what "the voices" are saying to him. He reports that he hears unrecognized voices laughing at him and calling him a "queer." He has the delusion that unnamed "foreigners" have a special mission for him that will make his name recognized by millions of people for hundreds of years. The patient repeatedly tells about his nose having been broken two years ago, implying that his current situation is somehow related to that event. Other content of thought includes themes of current confusion, difficulty with decisions, preoccupation with sexual matters, and bewilderment about his future. The patient denies suicidal thought. Impaired judgment is evidenced by his statement that if he found an addressed envelope with an uncanceled stamp, he would take it to the chief of police. The patient shows impaired abstracting ability on testing with both proverbs and similarities. Although the patient has some insight into the fact that all is not well in his life and that he should take prescribed medication, he specifically denies that he has any mental problem.

7

Closing the Interview

After the opening of the interview and a period of mutual exploration, there needs to be some form of closing, which both doctor and patient should anticipate. In starting a relationship with a psychiatric patient, or any patient, it is reassuring to the patient if the doctor gives him or her some idea of the limits and bounds of that relationship. This does not mean that you should force the patient into a rigid time schedule, but the doctor needs to plan ahead, and the patient will feel better if he or she has some idea of what to expect. In the beginning, therefore, it is best to let the patient know about how much time there will be for this and subsequent interviews and what will take place during the interviews. You may not want to state a definite amount of time at first, but comments such as "We have time. Tell me more about it," give the patient a general idea of the available time. At the first contact with a patient, one might say "I'd like to hear about your problems and learn more about you, and after that we will do a physical exam."

Interviews should never go to the point of exhaustion for both parties. One hour is a good length for an individual interview, but much can be accomplished with a shorter interview. One and one-half hours can be productive for the initial interview. Toward the end of the interview, the doctor should say "Our time is about up" or "We have about five minutes left." This gives patients a chance to regroup and to add other things that they may not have mentioned yet.

Don't feel bad about ending an interview. You can always come back. If something seemingly important is brought up at the end, you can say "We will have to stop, but perhaps you would like to talk about that next time."

Sometimes the doctor gives the patient a short summary of what has taken place in the interview, but this is not always necessary. Whether or not to summarize at the end of each interview is something to be judged with each patient. Since the summary will inevitably be weighted toward what the interviewer believes to be important, it helps the patient to understand what the doctor is looking for. On the other hand, a summary may not always be desirable because the patient will come to depend on it and slant the interview too much toward what the doctor wants.

Closing is not difficult, particularly if the doctor does not feel guilty about it. Patients like to feel that the time spent together was somewhat productive and mostly it is. Certainly no one solves all their problems in one interview. A statement such as "Well, we got a little more understanding of your past life today" can give a patient a good feeling without promising too much.

Sometimes a patient will say, "Well, doctor, now that I've told you all this, what do you think?" There is a great temptation to answer this question at the end of the interview, particularly if you make some sense out of what the patient has said and can put together some hypotheses about why their situation is as it is. We should resist the temptation to pontificate.

I have said these two things before, but they are worth repeating. Nothing is as simple as it seems, and the insights of the most help to a patient are his or her own. As I have noted in earlier examples of interviews, you can say "After having reviewed some of your life, what do you think?" Or, if this doesn't work or doesn't seem appropriate, you can say "I'm not going to be able to give you the answer, but I am willing to help you work on these problems, and maybe together we can help you figure out how to do things differently." There are many different ways to communicate that the interview or interviews are a shared experience, that the doctor will help all he or she can, but the patient must also take responsibility and the doctor will try to help the patient learn from the experience.

The question "What do you think, doctor?" is a reasonable question for any patient to ask; however, the interviewer should be aware that such a question may also be a final attempt to see if the doctor won't relent, let the patient be dependent, and give him or her the answer. Psychiatrists sometimes clarify these thoughts for their patients by saying something such as "You may think I have all of the answers and for some reason I'm just not telling you. I wish I did have the answer, but I don't; however, I am willing to help you try to work things out."

Many patients do not ask for anything at the end of an interview. They feel relieved by having someone listen to them and by being able to express some of their feelings. This probably is true with most patients and they need no closing statement about what might have happened in the interview.

Patients do need some idea about what will happen next, whatever it is. If this is the last interview, there should be some discussion of that. If there will be more, you should discuss when the patient will see you again and what else might happen.

A final element to closing is a little more subtle and intangible. The entire doctor–patient encounter has its opening, middle phase, and closing, and the same is true for each interview. We have already discussed starting and the body of the interview. If the patient, as well as the doctor, knows when the interview will be closing, then the tone will change toward the end and both will prepare themselves for leaving by not opening major new topics, but reflecting on what was said, or thinking about future appointments.

Some patients, because of dependency needs or anxiety, or both, will attempt to hold on to the doctor and prolong the interview. There are many ways to do this. Some simply continue to talk. Others will bring up a new and apparently important subject at the end. A few will say "But doctor, you haven't told me anything. You haven't helped me or given me any medicine." These patients want something more tangible. Since you don't have all of the answers, sometimes the most tangible thing you can offer is the next appointment.

Leaving a Service

Students, during the course of their medical school education and later as residents in training, find themselves leaving a particular service and, thus, they must terminate their relationships with patients. After a 6- to 8-week rotation on a service, students may find they have developed a fairly intense relationship with a patient whom they have been following in therapy. Although students might want to, they cannot continue this relationship, due to the demands of the next service to which they will be rotating. Students will probably have strong feelings about this termination and, most certainly, patients will have some feelings about it. These will be more intense than the feelings involved in closing a single interview.

Just as in closing a single interview, the termination should be anticipated and discussed ahead of time. It should not be left until the last interview to tell the patient that the student and patient will not be meeting again. The patient must have some time to work out feelings about termination or about the loss of the therapist. A general rule is that the more intense the therapeutic relationship has been and the more times the patient has been seen, the longer the period allowed for terminating the relationship should be. For example, if a student starts with a patient in the inpatient service, the emergency room, or the outpatient service in the first week of an 8-week clerkship and meets with him or her one or more times per week, then the patient should know fairly early in that relationship that it is limited. The patient should be reminded of termination again in the next to the last visit.

At this point, the student can ask the patient how he or she feels about not being able to see the student again for therapy. Patients' responses to this question vary. Most will start out by saying "Oh, I understand that you will be going on to another service and will be too busy to see me." Usually the patient will stop with such a remark. The student might then say "Well, even though you understand, maybe you have some feelings about my not being able to see you again." Usually the patient will say something to the effect that they are going to miss the student or they've enjoyed working with them. Patients do not easily express the anger that they feel about being abandoned. The student can respond by saying "Well, I have enjoyed seeing you" or "I hope it has been helpful to you for us to work together," and then add "But, I wonder if you are not a bit irritated or upset because you cannot continue coming in to see me." Most patients are angry about the termination because they feel that they're being abandoned. Usually they are not willing to express the anger unless given permission. Some patients may not even express their anger then. There are, of course, a few patients who are not angry. If the patient's hostility can be expressed, then the termination can be much more constructive. The patient can learn that it is all right to be angry with someone who has tried to help them.

No matter what the reason for termination, and no matter how well patients understand this, they are likely to have fantasies about why they're no longer being followed by the same student. Usually the patient will think that the student is leaving because he or she doesn't like the patient or that the student has more interesting patients to see. The patient may feel unworthy of the student's attention and see that as the reason for termination. Patients often have fantasies centered around their hostility towards the termination. These may take the form of fearing that something will happen to the therapist, such as an accident. These irrational fantasies exist along with a patient's rational understanding of the situation. A patient with a great deal of insight might say, "Well, I understand that you are going to another service and this really doesn't have anything to do with me, but I can't help feeling that the main reason you don't want to see me is that I am such a shallow person, that I am not interesting to you."

Students also have feelings about having to leave their patients. They may experience some sadness or depression about the loss of a relationship, or they may find themselves getting unreasonably angry just as the patient might do. The student's reaction is almost always far less intense than the patient's.

8

How to Handle Some
Special Problems

The student should learn a standard method of interviewing and then how to vary this according to the needs of each patient. First, learn some basic principles, learn how to apply them, and then learn the exceptions. This gives one a comfortable base, not to stand pat on, but to move to and from as the need arises. The nondirective approach, begun as an entree to mutual exploration by doctor and patient of the patient's emotional and psychological states and past history, is a basic foundation from which to advance to more specialized techniques. From a nondirective beginning, you can easily become more directive, more reassuring, or more concrete as the need arises. And the need does frequently arise.

One of the intriguing and stimulating aspects of medicine is that no two patients are alike. Nowhere are differences more apparent than when you work in the area of personality and interpersonal interactions. There cannot be too many hard and fast rules about the doctor–patient interaction. Flexibility is most important, coupled with an ability to appraise the emotional climate of an interaction quickly and to modify your approach accordingly. Many people, of course, can do this intuitively, but everyone benefits by learning and practice.

As physicians, we strive to make our intuition explicit, our information as scientifically accurate as possible, and, it goes without saying, to use what we know for the patient's benefit. Therefore, as early as possible in the interview the physician should begin to formulate a hypothesis about how the patient is feeling and reacting to this interview. One can then test out the hypothesis by verbal or nonverbal intervention and modify one's approach accordingly.

I will discuss some common problems here which, when encountered in interviewing, call for modification of the nondirective exploration of a patient's state of mind. Doggedly pursuing a nondirective approach with some of the kinds of patients mentioned here could easily heighten the already incapacitating level of feelings present or, in patients with intellectual impairment, lead to needless frustration.

People have different ways of responding to stress and illness. The response is determined by a complex interaction of biologic propensities (which we often call temperament), past interpersonal interactions (the importance of childhood history), and the present situation. Individual reaction is almost as varied as people, but reactions do fall into some general types. I will cover some of these as well as how to vary the interview technique to help the patient cope with sometimes overpowering feelings.

The physician should not make a moral judgment about whether one response pattern is superior to another. One response may be better than another for a certain patient's well-being, but the interviewing physician realizes that the patient's response is a complex biopsychosocial phenomenon to be understood, not to be judged on moral grounds. The physician's own emotional reaction to the patient is to be understood in the same light and used as data, not judged to be good or bad. Feel, empathize, understand, but at the same time be objective about emotions.

The Anxious Patient

Anxiety is ubiquitous. We have already discussed putting the patient at ease and, because all patients have some anxiety almost all of the time, it is always necessary, and should become automatic, to make comments or in some way help to relieve normal anxiety. Normal anxiety, however, is usually not incapacitating and may even be a stimulus to superior performance, as with athletes and actors.

Some patients' anxiety in the interview is great enough to be incapacitating. These patients need special help to feel more comfortable and enter into the interaction of the interview. Certain patients may never achieve this degree of comfort, but most can and there are ways of helping to reduce the anxiety. There are also ways of increasing the anxiety in a patient and these you want to avoid. Ignoring anxiety is a common fault among physicians and may serve to increase the level of feeling in both doctor and patient.

As anxiety begets anxiety, the interviewer must be at least minimally comfortable while interviewing. This doesn't mean free of anxiety. Students will have a lot of anxiety and anxiety will crop up from time to time all through your professional life. If students are aware of their anxiety, they can control it better and realize that it need not interfere too much with the relationship with the patient.

Before discussing some ways of relieving a patient's anxiety, we should say something about anxiety itself. Anxiety and fear have identical manifestations. Fear is defined as a response to a real danger. The feeling you have seeing an automobile coming toward you on the wrong side of a superhighway is fear. Anxiety, although having the same physiologic response, is defined as the fear of an imagined threat. Anxiety can be diffuse or specific. With diffuse anxiety, we feel anxious but do not know why. There is a reason or reasons for the fear, but for the moment we are unaware of those reasons. Diffuse anxiety can occur in anyone at most any time: when you are reading this book, for example. It may relate back to uncomfortable, traumatic, repressed feelings and experiences. Some anxiety has a biological component which, of course, must be investigated.

Mr. A, the patient who was born in England during the war, says, "I just start walking. I don't know why," and he tells us he has to take a drink before going to the store. We have discussed the many roots of his anxiety: the war, being deserted by his mother, anger at his mother for her alcoholism, fear that the anger would get out of control, and the possibility of a biological component such as in panic disorder. However, he had not been aware of the causes of this anxiety in the past.

Specific anxiety relates to something a person is afraid of, but knows there is no reason to be afraid. These are phobias that usually also have repressed traumatic experiences behind them, but are attached to a specific thing. Fear of the dark is a common example. Unless you are walking down a dark street where muggings occur frequently, there is probably little reason to fear the dark. What does it mean? It means different things for different people, but for some it may date back to a fear that our mother would not come at night when we needed her.

Now that we know reasonable people can have unreasonable fears when they see their doctor, what do we do about it? Most patients' fears are alleviated as we mentioned in "Starting the Relationship." If these do not help a patient feel comfortable enough for him or her to begin to enter into the interview, we must do more. With the young man who wanted to know what he would be expected to talk about, the interviewer was more active at the beginning of the interview, allowing the patient some more time to settle in and relax. For him, this was adequate, but for the interview we report later in the "Epilogue," even more specific questions were necessary.

Some interviews must start as directive interviews, with specific questions being asked, or the uncertainty aroused will be incapacitating to an anxiety-prone patient. The problem is then how to move from a directive to a nondirective approach. Carrying on a directive interview too long crystalizes the patient in a dependent position, waiting for questions to answer. When the doctor finally runs out of questions, the interview is over.

A few direct questions and an explanation of what the interview is about may suffice to relieve the anxiety. One can determine this simply by throwing in a nondirective question such as, "Now that I've asked you some questions and told you what we will be doing here today, why don't you tell me more about the problems that brought you here?" If the patient is still not able to enter into the interview, the next step is to comment on the anxiety. One can simply say "You seem worried" or "You seem to be afraid. Are you still worried about what might happen here?" After such a statement, the doctor waits for a response, which he or she and the patient might discuss. After this the doctor should indeed explain more about what is going to happen. That is, "We are just going to talk today. I'd like to find out more about you and something about your past life" or "We will talk and then I'll do a physical examination," or whatever.

Again, if this doesn't suffice, one should take additional steps to try to relieve the anxiety. This means making some attempt to identify the causes—not the early childhood causes, but some more recent causes—which may indeed derive from early childhood experiences. One statement could be "Are you worried about what we will talk about?" Then the doctor can pause a moment for the patient to respond. Depending on the response, he or she might then say "Maybe you're afraid I'll ask you some embarrassing questions." Then one can go on to reassure patients that they do not need to talk about anything they do not want to talk about.

Many patients who come for a psychiatric evaluation are afraid that they are crazy and will be locked up. Most patients know little about mental illness and have many unreasonable fears about it. This fear can be dealt with directly and the patient can be reassured. Start with a simple question such as, "Are you afraid that we are going to find that you are crazy?" or "Some people are afraid to come to a psychiatric clinic because they are afraid the doctor might think that they are crazy and lock them up. Have you been afraid of that?"

After the patient responds to such questions, it is important to give factual information and reassurance. Some patients may need to be hospitalized for their mental illness, but this is different from being "locked up." It is like being hospitalized for any other illness and most times patients are out of the hospital after a short stay and can resume their usual activities. Also, patients can be reassured that many people come to psychiatrists because they have problems and that doesn't mean that they are "crazy." Sometimes it may be helpful to ask the patient what he or she means by "crazy."

After going through this or a similar series of steps to help patients deal with their anxiety, we find with some patients that the anxiety level is still so high as to present a serious barrier to communication. Such anxiety may not diminish for several interviews.

With patients who have high anxiety, one must continue to use a more directive interview. Sitting silently waiting for a frightened patient to respond only adds to the tension; therefore, the first interview with these patients may well be a series of direct questions with the patient replying with short answers. I do not prefer this type of interview, but it is possible, although difficult, for one or more such interviews to be a prelude to a more open-ended discussion with the patient. The doctor should not overlook this possibility.

PANIC STATES

Anxiety may progress to panic. In panic the anxiety is so acute that it leads to personality disorganization. The patient may present with extreme restlessness, pacing, weeping, and may seem unable to talk or listen. Panic states are usually seen in the emergency room. When confronted with a patient in panic, the interviewer must be especially empathic, supportive, and more direct in communication. First, openly recognize that the patient is in the grip of tremendous fear. Then tell the patient that you will be able to help and reassure him or her that talking about fears will help.

The interview is best conducted in a quiet room. Allow the patient to go into the room, or if the patient is already in the room when the interviewer enters, the interviewer should ask the patient's permission to close the door. Some patients are fearful about being in a closed room. If so, the door should be left open. If someone has brought the patient in and the patient seems to gain support from that person, then invite him or her into the interview room. You must quickly and astutely evaluate the relationship and first ask the patient if he or she approves of the person being present during the interview. The clinician can say "Would it be helpful to you to have _____ in here with us?" If no one has come with the patient, it may be advisable to have a nurse or another supportive person in the room during the interview.

Some patients in panic like a feeling of closeness and reassurance, but many will not, and until this is determined, allow the patient some space. Do not intrude on his or her personal space until you determine that this will not increase the panic. It is best not to touch the patient. You do not know the patient and do not know how touching will be received. In this situation, the clinician must be even more careful to monitor his or her own body language. The doctor should not suggest withdrawal by leaning back in the chair but, rather, show attention by leaning forward, yet not intruding on the patient's personal space.

Some patients cannot sit still. If so, they should be allowed to move around the room.

The clinician must impart a feeling of confidence, because his or her anxiety will only serve to increase the patient's panic. Another person in the room helps support the interviewer as well as the patient. More than at any other time, patience on the part of the interviewer is most important. A voice with a lack of urgency or hesitancy will do much to reduce the panic state. The interviewer must also tell patients that they can be helped, that no one will hurt them, and that they will be protected.

In this reassuring situation, the interviewer, often with the help of a third party, attempts to get the patient to discuss fears. Sometimes the interviewer must talk a lot and ask questions. Confronted with this, the nondirective approach may be tried, but it should be quickly abandoned if it does not produce results.

The Hostile Patient

As anxiety begets anxiety, hostility provokes hostility: as we have said before, emotions are contagious. The patient who is angry provokes anger in the doctor. The general rule again applies: doctors must first be aware of their own anger in order to deal with the anger in their patients. If you respond to the patient's anger with hostility, the patient will usually be provoked to greater hostility. Contrary to popular opinion, few psychiatric patients are dangerous. Almost all patients have sufficient control of hostility so as not to hurt or endanger another. Nevertheless, in an occasional patient, hostility may get out of control. These patients are most often encountered in the emergency room or on a psychiatry inpatient service. They may have been brought in against their will or they may have come voluntarily because of their own fear of their violent impulses. Violence may occur in patients with a number of possible diagnoses. Occasionally, a delirious patient in a medical or surgical unit will have hostility that becomes out of control.

When encountering overt, threatening behavior, be calm and do not threaten the patient. Heroics have no place in these situations. If you have any reason to suspect that a patient's hostility may become out of control, let the patient know that he or she will not be allowed to hurt anyone and that he or she will be controlled if necessary. This information must be imparted in a reassuring, firm, but not hostile manner. The physician should also make sure that sufficient personnel are available to help control the patient. Most patients welcome such firm limits because of their great fear that they might act out their hostility.

Uncontrolled hostility can be a problem; however, we are also con-

cerned with hostility that threatens a constructive doctor–patient interaction. Taking a firm but nonthreatening attitude, while acknowledging some hostility on the part of the patient, will usually diminish
the hostility sufficiently to complete the interview. The doctor can say
"It sounds as if you are angry" or if the cause is known, "Maybe
you're a little upset about seeing a new doctor today."

It is best, when commenting on it, to understate the anger. Patients
are usually reluctant to acknowledge their anger to those in authority,
but they may be willing to admit some irritation. The patient might
start by admitting that things are not quite as they would wish, for
example, that they would prefer to have seen the doctor they saw last
week. Allowing the patient to express this may be all that is necessary
to relieve tension so that the interview may proceed. At other times,
the doctor can move from helping the patient express a little irritation
to expressing downright anger. This is usually therapeutic if the doctor
can accept the anger.

The following illustrates how a hostile patient provoked hostility in
a medical student. This student was aware of his hostility and attempted
to control it. The interview is with a 41-year-old man who was referred
to the medicine clinic after coming to the emergency room with complaints of severe nausea and vomiting of two days' duration. The material is presented in the student's own words.

I had to call the man's name four or five times before he came forward. As
the man walked past me through the door I could tell that he was probably an
alcoholic as he reeked of alcohol, walked rather wobbly, and was emaciated.

I introduced myself and asked "What seems to be the matter?" After a
short period of silence, during which time I glanced over the form of humanity
sitting before me and, while wondering how in the world a man can abuse his
body like he had, the patient burst forth with, "Well, to start off with, I have
been here for four hours waiting to be seen after staying in the emergency
room all morning; for all you people care a guy could die waiting out in front!"
To this I reacted rather hostilely and said, "Now wait just a minute; I realize
that you may have a reason to be angry, but I just work here and there is no
reason why you should take it out on me. I am here to help you if I can, and
if you want to cooperate, I'll do all I can." Reluctantly the patient straightened
his head up from a bowed position and said, "Well, doctor, I have been sick
at my stomach and vomiting for the past two days. I feel as if I am gonna die,
just like I told those doctors in the emergency room, but they would not give
me anything."

Feeling still rather hostile, I said, "Have you been drinking?" To this he
meekly nodded in the affirmative and said, "For the past two weeks I have
drunk a lot of wine, but not any of that whiskey." I said, "Have you been
drunk for that long, and when is the last time you had anything to eat?" [two
questions at once]. He answered, "I have been drunk for the last week and
haven't ate anything since Sunday." Well, at this point I was about to explode,

so I turned and walked out of the room before I said something that I should not have said. I remained out of the room while I talked this over with myself, and finally came to the conclusion that I would never get anywhere with the man unless I kept control of myself [the importance of being aware of one's feelings]. After a few minutes I returned to the room aware that I was halfway hoping that he had left. I found him lying on the table looking like death warmed over. I took about 15 minutes to try and explain to him the evils of alcohol and threw a good scare into him. [Let's see if this advice is of any value to the patient.] This seemed to bring him to his senses, and throughout the remainder of the interview he was very cooperative. I was feeling better and had my hostility in check until he volunteered that he had been a diabetic for ten years, taking 20 units of insulin until two years ago. When I asked the reason for termination of insulin, he replied that he did not have the money to purchase the insulin and the wine too, so he just bought the wine. This renewed my hostility toward the patient because of the "don't care" attitude he was taking. Somehow I managed to control myself and tried to explain to the patient the dangers that this entailed, to which he sat and listened attentively.

After consulting with the attending staff person, it was decided to give the patient some antacids, do the routine procedures for diabetic workup, and send him to the diabetic clinic. So I returned to the patient and took great care in explaining the procedures which he was to do before going to the diabetic clinic the next Wednesday, thinking all the time that he would probably do exactly what he wanted to do, although he appeared interested. When the patient left the room, he thanked me for what I had told him and appeared to have lost his hostility which he had when he first entered the room. I said to myself, "I sure hope he follows instructions."

The following Monday morning I ran into him in the elevator and on questioning him, learned that he had done just what I suspected—just what he wanted to do. He did not do anything that I had instructed him to do except come to the hospital for a FBS [fasting blood sugar].

It is this type of patient that not only brings out the hostility in a medical student but also in almost any practicing physician. The patient at the onset appeared to be hostile because of having to wait so long before being seen. When confronted with his rather "don't care" attitude, he became very passive and gave the impression that he didn't care if anything was done for him. Also, it was very perplexing to attempt to treat a patient that one could not trust to carry out instructions. I have seen several of this type of patient but, I must say, this one brought out my hostility more than any of the others.

The fact that this student was aware of his hostility was positive. More experience in medicine might lessen the hostility and engender greater acceptance of patients with diverse backgrounds. But physicians cannot and should not be devoid of feelings, nor should they repress their feelings. Only by becoming more aware and developing more understanding of feelings can the doctor react more therapeutically to patients.

The Patient Who Won't Talk

Because of anxiety, hostility, or other reasons, some patients are unable to talk. In the worst cases, this takes the form of no speech at all with perhaps an occasional nod or a "yes" or "no." Others will talk by giving specific answers to questions, but will volunteer little or no information. This is better than not talking at all, but it does severely limit what the patient and the doctor can obtain from their interaction.

The general principles I have stated before also apply to handling this situation. First, the interviewer must be aware of his or her own reaction to this behavior by the patient. Usually, the patient who is not complying and is being negativistic will provoke anxiety and hostility in the examiner because the examiner is not getting the information he or she needs to help the patient. Being aware of his or her own feelings, the physician is less likely to act impulsively on them.

The next step is to take the means already discussed to relieve the patient's anxiety. If hostility is the main problem, it may be necessary to comment on this. If the patient is still unresponsive, several other avenues are open. You can terminate the interview and try again another time. If the interview is terminated, let the patient know that the doctor is still interested in him and will continue to try to help him or her. A statement to this effect is helpful, "It seems to be hard for you to talk with me now. Perhaps coming into the hospital (or whatever) is too upsetting for you to talk now. I still want to get to know you and do all I can to help you. We can stop for now, but I will be back this afternoon (or tomorrow) and we can start again."

Another approach is for the doctor to talk more. This is contrary to my previous advocacy of minimum action on the part of the doctor. However, it may be supportive for a patient who is unable to talk to be relieved of the burden of producing something for the doctor. In this situation, the doctor can start by making a few remarks about what is known about the patient and then asking a question. If there is no response, you can talk more about patients' anxiety and how it is hard to share one's inner feelings with strangers. If all of this fails, you might talk about neutral subjects while watching the patient's response.

A third course, if the previous attempts have failed, is to sit silently with the patient for a few minutes, making a comment now and then. Silence must be used carefully and only if the physician is comfortable and the patient appears not too anxious, because silence tends to increase, rather than decrease, anxiety.

With patients who do not talk, nonverbal responses become especially important. The examiner should watch facial expressions and body movement. These may show whether the patient is comprehending what is being said, and whether he or she is being attentive or even purposely inattentive.

The Rambling, Circumstantial, Overly Talkative Patient

The rambling, circumstantial, or overly talkative patient may be at first a welcome relief for someone who is learning interviewing. At last, a patient who will talk and one need only sit back and listen! Soon, however, the interviewer begins to worry about having enough time to get a satisfactory history of the present illness. Forget the past history for today. This is the patient who may have first developed pains in the back of her neck about six months ago. As a matter of fact, it was about the time of her niece's wedding. A nice young girl and that boy she married—well, his family were not much to look at, but the father. . . .

On and on it goes, sometimes an interesting story, but much of it not relevant. This is another exception to the general rule of allowing the patient to tell the story his or her own way. Most of the time what comes out is important and it may also be with the overly talkative patient. With this patient, however, the important information may be obscured or deliberately, if unconsciously, hidden by details and tangential verbal excursions.

Sometimes if these patients are allowed to talk on for a reasonable period of time they will slow down and the interview may proceed as usual; however, this does not always happen and they must be interrupted. You might interrupt any patient occasionally, but an interview with the overly talkative patient is one of the few occasions when the interviewer will need to interrupt a patient repeatedly. The rambling patient must be brought back to the topic at hand, if possible.

The Dependent Patient

Dependency and the tendency to regress to earlier behavior patterns are universal responses to illness. When they come to see the doctor, all patients will show some signs of what we could call dependent behavior. Looking for clues as to what to do and asking advice about their problems are signs of normal dependency. Some patients are overly dependent and either show this directly or they react against their dependency by the opposite behavior: being overly independent.

The excessively dependent patient may appear overly eager to please or be openly demanding. These patients, in one way or another, show that they want to be taken care of. They often have unreal expectations about what their doctor can or is willing to do for them, and whatever is done is usually not enough (Kahana and Bibring 1964). According to the developmental theory of emotional development, these characteristics are a carryover from unmet dependency needs during infancy. Ideally, we would help the patient discuss his or her exaggerated need to be taken care of and why this came about. With most excessively dependent patients this is not possible, although one might occasionally suggest discussion of this.

Much has been written about patients who come back again and again with the same problems or, if they get rid of one problem have another. A doctor feels angry and frustrated about a patient whom he or she cannot help. The key to working with these patients is not giving in to one's own frustrations while also not completely giving in to the patient's dependency. These patients need a doctor whom they can count on, one who will see them, listen to their complaints and, within reasonable limits, try to alleviate their suffering, and be there when they return. Some of the dependency needs must be met while maintaining realistic limits on the doctor–patient relationship and the treatment given.

One thing young doctors must soon learn is that they cannot like everyone who comes in to see them. Some people will appeal to them more than others, and it will sometimes be hard to find something likable about certain patients. Inasmuch as doctors, as well as patients, have different personalities, their likes and dislikes will be different. Some will feel the most hostility toward anxious patients. Other doctors will find themselves becoming unduly anxious when a patient expresses any hostility. For still others, the dependent, clinging patient who does not seem to be motivated to do anything and who never seems to get entirely well, is the bane of their existence.

A 72-year-old man was complaining to a student about the pains in his joints. He said he had not been doing well since his last clinic visit and wondered if the student was really helping him. The patient said, "I got home last week and got to wondering if you were old enough to know what you are doing."

The patient then went on to say that his wife didn't take him seriously either (implying that the student didn't take the man's complaints seriously).

The patient then said, "Doc, can't you see I'm a sick man? Why, I remember when I was young and used to get sick, Ma used to wait on me hand and foot. It didn't take long for me to get well then. What's wrong with people today?"

As the patient had no serious physical illness, he was reassured by the student, but, following this reassurance, he complained of a new pain in his shoulder. After that he said, "Doc, I've always been a person who needs a little help now and then. I remember I used to depend on Ma to help me. Mama used to help me, but lately she just fusses and fumes everytime I want something. I get upset because I can't get no help. Doc, ain't you going to help me?"

The student again tried to reassure the man by telling him that he had had a thorough examination, with all the necessary tests, and it showed that he was in good health. In spite of this, the patient left looking forlorn and grumbling about his joints.

The next week the patient returned looking happy and stated that he was much improved. "Doc, I got to thinking you probably know more than I gave you credit for. Yessiree, I'm lots better—even played dominoes with the boys last week. You know, Mama and me have been getting along much better. Why she started looking after me and even told me I was almost getting romantic again."

Was it the student's reassurance or Mama's attention that made the patient feel better?

The Suicidal Patient

An interview with a patient who has attempted suicide or is believed to be suicidal is apt to be strained and unproductive if the suicidal attempts or thoughts are not acknowledged early in the interview. Some interviewers are fearful about bringing up the subject of suicide, as if mentioning suicide might increase its likelihood. On the contrary, most patients are willing to discuss their suicidal thoughts and may even be relieved to be asked about them.

For a patient who has not attempted suicide, but in whom suicidal thoughts are suspected, begin exploration by asking about depression: "Have you been feeling depressed lately?" The depression can be explored along with sleep patterns and other vegetative signs of depression, possible precipitating circumstances, and past episodes. It is simple, somewhere in the course of the exploration, to say, "Have you felt so depressed that you have considered ending it all?"

Suicidal thoughts can then be discussed. One should ask if there have been actual plans for suicide. If so, you must assess their lethality and the patient's knowledge of their lethality. A person who has bought a gun and bullets and picked a time for suicide is in great danger. If he or she has made a will and given away possessions, the danger is even greater.

The interviewer will usually find that most patients have not taken such extreme steps. No matter how preliminary or tentative, all suicidal thoughts should be taken seriously and actively evaluated. Here again, the interviewer deviates from the nondirective approach and probes in order to gather necessary information.

It is important to interview the suicidal patient's family and significant others to learn about possible precipitating events, possible supportive individuals in their environment, and to assess recent changes in behavior.

The Patient with Concrete Thinking

Interviewing as discussed in this book presupposes a patient of average intelligence who is capable of abstract thinking and can express thoughts and experiences verbally. Only patients with this ability can respond as we would hope to such a question as, "What was it like while you were growing up?" Intelligence and abstracting ability do not necessarily correlate with education. Many of the patients whose interviews are mentioned in this book did not graduate from high school, but they are intelligent and readily grasp emotional and intellectual concepts.

Some patients, however, are unable to think abstractly and, if this is not recognized early, the interview becomes a frustrating experience for both patient and doctor. The inability of a patient to understand conceptually what the doctor has in mind is one reason why interviews flounder, even though the physician may be making the right statements, relieving the patient's anxiety, and otherwise conducting the interview properly.

The following is taken from an interview with a mildly retarded young man who was pleasant, cooperative, and very concrete in his thinking. His concreteness made it difficult to engage him at any length in exploring feelings about his interactions with significant people.

STUDENT: Well, Clyde, why don't you tell me something about yourself?

PATIENT: I'm 22 years old. I'm from Nashville, Tennessee. I'm working in the Around Town Janitor Services trying to be a janitor. That's about all.

STUDENT: Tell me about your family.

PATIENT: My grandmother's in Nashville. My mother's here. My little brother's working in a restaurant.

STUDENT: How are you making it financially?

PATIENT: As best I can.

STUDENT: Well, how do you do that?

PATIENT: Like I say, I'm trying to get a job as a janitor.

STUDENT: Tell me about things you do for fun.

PATIENT: I go to ball parks, play ball, draw pictures, and things like that.

(Interview continues like this for a while.)

STUDENT: Is there anything you'd like to tell me about yourself?

PATIENT: When I was growing up I wasn't around people. Now I am, and I'm learning to handle my own problem.

STUDENT: What is your problem?

PATIENT: People tried to run over me, but now I can handle it.

STUDENT: Talking about your marriage?

PATIENT: Went downhill all the way.

STUDENT: How?

PATIENT: Well, one night I went to bed and two cops came and knocked at the door and took my brother to jail. She said he was wrecking the marriage. I had to get dressed and go bail him out, and after that it was downhill all the way.

STUDENT: What kind of work did you do in Nashville?

PATIENT: Dishwasher.

STUDENT: How did you like it?

PATIENT: Fine; hard work but good money.

STUDENT: What kind of people would you admire?

PATIENT: What do you mean?

STUDENT: Strong kind or what?

PATIENT: Like my wife, she didn't clean house.

STUDENT: Tell me about your grandmother.

PATIENT: She's 74 years old. She's got her house. She's got a garden, plants, stuff in the garden. (pauses)

STUDENT: Did you get along well with her?

PATIENT: Yes, I did.

STUDENT: What about your school?

PATIENT: Well, I'm a slow learner, so I was held back.

The patient's response to "Tell me about your grandmother" is probably the most vivid example of his concrete thinking. There were no abstractions in the interview. Even when he was telling about his relationship with his wife, the patient explained it in terms of a specific event. This man was doing the best he could. It was not emotions such as anxiety or hostility that prevented a more elaborate response, it was limitation of intelligence.

Patients with organic brain disorders and mental retardation will show concrete thinking. Once it is recognized, the cause must be determined. Some patients with normal or low/normal intelligence have a limited ability to understand their own feelings. These patients may need to be interviewed in a more direct way, with special attention to whether or not they understand what they are being asked.

Crying

We expect to see crying on television and in the movies, but in other situations it is often distressing to the person crying and to those in the immediate vicinity. An automatic response is to try to ignore the crying and change the subject that appeared to induce it.

Crying frequently occurs in psychiatric and other medical interviews and has a number of causes. Depression and sadness are the most obvious reasons, and are probably the most frequent causes. We can readily determine this from the content and feeling tone of the discussion. The best way to handle this kind of crying is to remain silent until the patient is under control, then comment that the patient is upset and suggest that he or she might want to talk more about these feelings. Patients will usually accept the opportunity to do this and will feel better. Occasionally, a patient will want to change the subject to gain better control, and, if so, he or she should be allowed to do so.

People cry for reasons other than sadness, and the interviewer should not always assume the person crying is sad. As one gains more experience, one learns to ask, "Why are you crying?" The answer is sometimes surprising. Many people, and especially women, cry when they are angry. If the interviewer is not aware of this, he or she will respond in a supportive manner as if the patient were sad and will miss what the patient is trying to express. Patients who cry in anger are often relieved just by expressing the feeling or need only verbal or nonverbal permission to express anger. I have had patients say, "Don't worry about me. I'm okay. I just cry when I'm mad."

Less commonly, patients will shed tears of joy or cry when they are frustrated. In either case, let them know that when they visit their doctor, it is all right to cry if they need to. You will rarely find a patient who abuses this privilege.

Answering Questions and Giving Advice

Patients come to doctors for answers to their questions and solutions to their health problems. Doctors realize this and, if they cannot fulfill their patients' expectations, they tend to feel inadequate. To avoid feeling inadequate and because we like the feeling of omnipotence brought by being sought out for advice, we tend to answer questions and give advice when asked, or sometimes when not asked. So, when a patient says, "Doctor, what do you think I should do?" we tend to respond by telling him or her what we think. To paraphrase an old saying, "Humans are never at a loss for opinions." Patients who ask their doctors for an opinion about what to do with their lives have probably received at least a dozen opinions on the same subject from friends, relatives, and their minister. That they ask for still another opinion may mean that they are not yet ready to solve their problem, and they hope that the doctor may finally provide an easy answer.

One of the most difficult tasks is to give good advice. It is even more difficult for the person receiving the advice to follow it. Hence, advice should be given sparingly, if at all.

Michael Balint says, "So the first principle should be: *Never advise or reassure a patient before you have found out what the real problem is.* More often than not, after the real problem has been brought to light, the patient will be able to solve it without the doctor's advice and reassurance" (Balint 1957).

You will recall when Mr. A said, "Why should it come out now?" the doctor responded by saying, "What do you think?" and Mr. A went right on with his analysis. Most patients are willing to try to work out the answers themselves if encouraged and helped to do so. The solutions patients work out have much more meaning for them and they are more apt to act on them.

As with all rules, there are exceptions. Some patients are so anxious and disorganized that they need specific advice to handle an immediate situation until they are well-enough organized to develop a long-term solution. For example, when a man comes in and says his four-year-old child is crying all the time and unable to sleep at night because the child is being abused during the day by its alcoholic mother, it is all right to say, "What do you propose to do about it?" If the husband says "I don't know—I'm so upset I can't think," then it is quite proper for the doctor to suggest an alternate care arrangement for the child. The doctor does not say "Divorce your wife." He or she merely offers the patient a way to cope with the acute situation. After this man solves his immediate problem, he will be better able to work towards a long-term solution.

Giving advice to a patient about how to live his or her life should always be the exception and not the rule. The rule is, as Dr. Balint says, explore and find the real problem.

The Forensic Examination

The interviewing discussed so far presupposes a cooperative, interested patient and a physician acting for and in the best interest of that patient. This technique, along with the nondirective approach and empathic ear, allows the physician to appreciate the patient's feelings. By gentle encouragement, the physician assists the patient in presenting material that will be of benefit to the physician in the evaluation and to the patient as he or she begins to understand some of his or her own thoughts and feelings. Even if the patient is initially an unwilling participant, such as a patient brought to the emergency room against his or her will by a relative, the physician usually can help put the patient at ease and eventually gain his or her confidence.

Physicians, especially psychiatrists, are sometimes called on by community agencies to examine a patient who may not have requested an examination. The physician may encounter an angry, hostile, uncooperative patient in the forensic psychiatric examination, where the physician is most often not the agent of the patient, but is called on by attorneys, the courts, the state, or others to make the examination.

In these instances, the physician is called on to give a professional opinion about the patient's mental health or illness, ability to tell right from wrong, to participate in the action called for, or other areas where lack of mental competence has been suspected. Patient and doctor frequently begin these encounters as adversaries, not in the friendly, supportive relationship that the patient would think to be to his or her benefit. The patient who sees the doctor in this way may not wish to participate and may resist the interview in a variety of ways.

Doctors tend to shy away from forensic interviews. Many would prefer not to get involved. Yet, the forensic interview is a necessary function and, at times, may prove to be in the patient's best interest. These interviews are necessary to determine competency to make a will, to marry, or to buy or sell property. Sometimes a psychiatrist is called in to determine the mental competency of an individual who refuses hospitalization or surgery that doctors have presented to the patient as necessary and perhaps even life saving. In these situations, the physician attempts to understand a patient's motivation for making his or her decision and determine whether this is based on rational judgment or distorted thinking produced by a mental illness.

The interview is one of the most important tools in making this determination. The forensic interview begins differently from what I have described in all of our other interviews. The physician must first advise the patient of his or her rights. The physician should introduce himself or herself, explain the purpose of the interview, and who requested it. The patient should be warned that the interview will not be confidential between doctor and patient, and that a report will be sent to whomever requested the information: perhaps a court, the district attorney, the patient's attorney, an opposing attorney, or a governmental agency. Prior to the start of the formal interview, it is advisable to have the patient sign a statement noting the nonconfidential nature of the interview.

The physician's opening statements impart a different feeling tone than in the interviews I have described. We have been discussing interviews in which the patient's welfare is the sole purpose and the patient decides how that will best be served. In the forensic interview, the patient has the right to decide how his or her welfare will best be served, but the interview is not necessarily for that purpose. After this initial encounter, however, an attempt is made to carry on an open-ended interview that allows patients to tell their story in their own way, as discussed above. This is not as easy in these situations, and you must, of necessity, evaluate the material somewhat differently. Patients are not apt to be as open and as honest when they know the interview will be reported to a third party as they are when they know that all the material is confidential and will only be used for their own benefit. This is particularly true in the evaluation of criminal behavior and when attempting to understand feelings, thoughts, and activities at the time the act was committed.

As they gain more understanding of the criminal behavior, examiners may be afraid that they will find material that may establish the patient's guilt. For this reason, he or she may be reluctant to carry out a thorough and intensive interview of all aspects of the possible unlawful acts or give a written evaluation of what was found. Nevertheless, this area is most important. From the legal point of view, it is necessary to evaluate the patient's state of mind at the time of the alleged criminal act. The physician, if he or she is aware of backing off from a thorough investigation, may be reminded that he or she is not a judge or jury. The physician does not make judgments or pass sentence, that is the province of the courts. His or her function in this particular interview is to gather information as thoroughly and scientifically as possible.

Taking this medical–legal position will no doubt create considerable conflict in many doctors and some will, perhaps correctly, choose not to be involved any more than is necessary. This is, of course, the physician's option and he or she should not hesitate to exercise it. Nevertheless, these examinations are important and, in some small way, the examiner may actually contribute to enlightening the legal system.

References

Balint M: *The Doctor, His Patient and the Illness*. New York, International Universities Press, 1957.

Kahana RJ, Bibring GL: Personality types in medical management, in Zinberg NE (ed): *Psychiatry in Medical Practice in a General Hospital*. New York, International Universities Press, 1964.

9

Some Common Pitfalls

Dealing with Events Instead of Feelings

The tendency to deal with facts to the exclusion of feelings has been mentioned before, but the problem is so common even among experienced interviewers that it merits further discussion. It is the unusual interviewer who does not need to combat consciously the automatic response to ask for specific external factual information about anything a patient says. Facts need to be recorded on the chart, they are usually easy to get, and patients expect to be asked about them.

A depressed woman says in the initial interview, "I have been married all of my adult life. My husband and I were childhood sweethearts, and after graduation from high school all I thought about was how great married life would be. But I found out differently."

The doctor then said, "How long have you been married?"

On hearing this question, one might think that the doctor did not want to know how the woman felt about her marriage. That may not have been so. It may simply have been easier and more customary to ask about the length of the marriage. Eventually, we need to know how long she has been married; however, a number of responses would have been more productive. A better response would have been either to say nothing and let the patient continue or, if she paused, to say something like, "What did you find out that was different?" Picking up her last words encourages continuation of her thoughts. Later, the interviewer can ask how long she has been married.

A rule to remember is that specifics of an event will often come out as a patient is asked about feelings, but feelings do not come forth as often when a patient is asked about events. If the woman had talked about the problems in her marriage, she may well have said something like, "In twelve years of marriage, we have done nothing but fight."

Now the doctor not only knows how long she was married, but he has much more information. Unless otherwise indicated, always opt to learn more about feelings when the opportunity is presented. You can always return to a subject to pick up a specific fact.

Asking More Than One Question at Once

Asking more than one question at once may be related to the interviewer's anxiety and need to talk, although it might be done in a well-meaning, but misguided, attempt to clarify for the patient what the physician is asking him or her.

A student interviewing a woman who brought her child to a pediatric clinic said, "Is everything going fine around your house? Everyone getting along well?"

An experienced psychiatrist, who should have known better, opened the interview with a patient being interviewed for a clinical teaching conference by saying, "We will be talking for a few minutes about some of your problems. You might start by telling me how you see your troubles. What brought you to the hospital?"

What brought the patient to the hospital and how he or she sees his or her troubles are not the same. One is an open-ended question and one is more specific. The doctor should not confuse the patient in the opening statement. By rehearsing statements in your mind before making them in the interview, you reduce the possibility of double questions.

Students, on learning to interview, often focus unduly on questions to be asked, thinking that the interview will rise or fall on their questions or that they must have all of their questions ready in order to keep the interview going. Some students say, "I ran out of questions so I had to stop." For these students, I say try to think of the interview as an interaction in which you, as the doctor, are encouraging the patient to go on talking about his or her problem. Rather than thinking of your next question, think of an encouraging remark or gesture. With this kind of interaction, the interview will unfold.

Answering the Question or Indicating the Preferred Answer

A woman said, "My husband worked at a meat packing plant, but he no longer works there." The interviewer asked, "Why did he stop? Was there no business?"

The statement, "Was there no business?" makes it hard for the patient to give another answer, such as he was fired. Patients are especially unlikely to give a negative answer if the physician indicates he or she wants a positive answer.

The question, "How are things going at home?" is a good one. If it is immediately followed by the second question, "Is everyone getting along well," the patient is apt to give little information. The doctor has already answered the question, or at least indicated the preferred answer. Patients rarely have the courage to contradict the doctor's predetermined outcome, even if things are not going well at home.

A patient who is reticent and fearful about expressing anger toward another will be relieved at the opportunity to agree with the psychiatrist who asks, "How are things going at work? Do you have a good boss?" A simple, "Yes, she's a good person" is a lot easier for this patient than saying, "My boss never appreciates how hard I work." Yet, the patient might have said that if the physician had stopped at, "How are things going at work?"

If an answer is supplied by an interviewer, it usually puts the patient in a positive light. This is done almost unconsciously to help relieve the patient's anxiety and thus some of the anxiety of the interviewer. The physician must listen to and critically evaluate every statement that comes from his or her own mouth.

Planning Ahead to the Next Question

The doctor must always have in mind where he or she needs to go in an interview, but this should be a general plan, the details to be filled in by the patient. Most of the doctor's actions during the interview should be in response to what the patient says and does at the time it occurs in the interview. The doctor moves in tune with the patient even though there are general goals in mind for the interview. Remember: relaxed attentiveness.

Many beginning interviewers are so worried about what they should say and do that they forget to listen. They are thinking about what to do and planning their next statement or question as the patient is talking. They then use what they planned whether or not it is appropriate to what the patient just said. Such interviewers are like a driver deciding he should turn after the next mile, but not bothering to see if the road turns where he wants to turn.

Becoming Overly Involved with the Patient

Psychoanalysts spend years trying to understand their feelings about their patients so as to avoid becoming emotionally involved in their patients' problems. All physicians should do likewise, albeit less formally. Every doctor does not need psychoanalysis, but every doctor should be wary of emotional involvement with patients.

The physician–patient relationship is a close one. A physician must be understanding, compassionate, and helpful to his or her patients. You can be most helpful by remaining objective. Patients, unless they are aloof from everyone, have no lack of compatriots who are entwined with them and their disturbed emotions. They don't need another one, least of all their physician.

Their emotional problems are compelling and it is tempting to try to step in and help straighten out the patient's life or to offer love and affection when the patient says no other exists. It's a fine line between empathy and sympathy, between respect and infatuation. Doctors are human, and all of their human emotions will, at one time or another, come to the fore as they practice. These emotions should be acknowledged and understood, but not acted upon.

The temptation to lose one's objectivity can occur with almost any patient. Each clinician, according to his or her own history, will find it more difficult to keep from being overly involved with particular patients. Adolescents, for example, can be appealing or, in some cases, the opposite if they are hostile, and so are apt to provoke strong positive or negative responses. Attractive patients of the opposite sex may invite emotional responses which should be acknowledged and controlled.

When a patient comes in and tells about how incompetent his or her last doctor was, listen but don't judge either the doctor or the patient. Acknowledge that the patient feels the way he or she does, but don't run out and try to settle matters with the previous doctor. Or, if a patient of the opposite sex tells how cold and callous his or her spouse is, don't admonish the spouse and certainly don't try to make up for that person's supposed deficiencies.

Being Taken In

Every one of us tends to report from our own point of view and we tend to report what makes us look most favorable. A person who is depressed or self-effacing will tend to overemphasize failure. We cannot always expect a patient to be objective; however, being objective and being honest are not always the same. A patient may feel that he or she is being honest, but emotions color perceptions and the patient's perceptions may not always agree with those of a more impartial observer. Of course, observers are not always impartial either, especially if they are family members.

No one wants to be made a fool of, and being taken in by an untrue story would seem intolerable for some. Yet this is bound to happen sooner or later as one deals with psychiatric patients—and probably sooner for the beginner. A patient may discuss a delusional system so logical that you cannot believe that the facts are not as the patient states them. It happens frequently when interviewing patients with antisocial personality disorder, who always minimize their wrong-doings so as to present themselves in the best light.

Physicians occasionally encounter the patient who presents with a factitious disorder. These patients fabricate physical complaints, inflict wounds upon themselves, or deliberately produce bleeding from an orifice, such as the ear or rectum. These patients have seen many physicians and have been hospitalized repeatedly. Although such extensive and deliberate lying is rarely seen, emotionally determined factual distortions are common.

To establish and foster the doctor–patient relationship, the interviewer should approach patients assuming they are doing their best to give a true picture of feelings and facts. Patients are anxious and fearful. Expressing doubts about their stories will only intensify the fear and anxiety and increase defensive measures, one of which is distortion. Establishing a relationship of mutual trust is primary, and the doctor must take the initiative here.

This does not mean that the interviewer accepts or believes everything the patient says. Maintaining an open mind is imperative. Occasionally, you might even ask the patient if there could be another interpretation, but always accept the patient's answer without pressing the matter. Do not be fearful about being taken in. It happens to the most experienced psychiatrists and will continue to occur if the doctor–patient relationship is the primary concern. As long as you maintain an open mind, the "real story," if there is one, will come forth. I say "if there is one" to remind the reader that emotions are also "real." You want more than "just the facts." If there are questions that can be answered by an interview with a family member or friend, such an interview is usually easily arranged. The common pitfall is that the clinician will be so concerned about getting a true story that he or she will ask entrapping questions or show distrust in other ways. If this happens, the kind of doctor–patient relationship that is conducive to mutual exploration will be impossible to develop.

Neglecting the Present Reality

After all I have said about psychological reality, I should add a word of caution about the "real" world outside. Patients do have environmental obstacles that are difficult to overcome. The clinician needs to know what they are and to be alert to their impact on therapy.

A 28-year-old man was being interviewed in a veterans' hospital.

He had been in the hospital three times before. At each time of discharge arrangements had been made for long-term follow-up outpatient treatment. The patient would keep one or two appointments but then fail to show up for others. Eventually, he would drop out of therapy and end up back in the hospital.

During the interview he was asked why he did not continue in outpatient treatment. He said,

> My family won't let me stay with them anymore. They say they can't control me. I've been living with a couple of buddies on the other side of town. We don't have any money. I've been selling my blood to the blood bank to get money, but have to use that for food and maybe a little beer sometimes. I don't have the money for the bus. The blood bank won't take me sometimes when my blood is down.
>
> I've tried to get a job, but I haven't worked for a long time. Employers will give me a chance, but they don't want someone who has to go to the doctor all the time. It got to be just too hard to come.

With some more effort, the man might have made all his appointments, but psychiatric patients are not always capable of such efforts. Furthermore, we all know that if there are some ambivalent feelings about coming, an outside obstacle can tip the scales against coming.

Environmental realities should be evaluated in an interview and patients need to be encouraged to talk about them. In psychiatry, you will find that most behavior is determined by what is going on inside the patient and by his or her perceptions of the outside world, but sometimes what is going on outside is a major detriment. The interviewer needs to find out about both.

10

Interviewing Significant Others and the Family

This book has been devoted almost entirely to the psychiatric interview of the individual patient. This is where most students begin and is the kind of psychiatric interviewing physicians will be doing during their professional lives. Family assessment is relatively new compared with diagnosis of an individual. Yet it adds an additional dimension to individual evaluation and treatment in many situations. Fine tuning the whole system—the family—may improve the function of each of the components. Sometimes the patient is not the most disturbed member of the family.

An older, apparently paranoid man came into the hospital complaining that his relatives were poisoning him so as to get his land—a familiar story given by a paranoid psychotic later in life. It turned out, however, that the relatives really were poisoning the man. What he perceived as happening was, in fact, happening.

Interviewing a significant other or the patient's family may not always give an objective point of view. Certainly, if a woman is putting arsenic in her husband's soup, she is not going to tell his doctor about it. (These situations do occur, and with one such patient, the diagnosis was not made until someone thought to do an analysis of the patient's hair.) Most often, however, interviewing others helps you to understand the patient's interpersonal relationships, those most helpful to recovery, and those needing some improvements.

Because psychiatric disorders occur in the context of interpersonal relationships, and because the relationships are principally in the family, clinicians should consider an interview with one or more family members as a part of every psychiatric evaluation. It is not necessary to interview a family member of every patient, but it should be considered. A family interview does not usually pose any difficulty because a relative of the patient will contact the patient's doctor. You should welcome this opportunity to learn more about the patient's problems.

Family interviews and family therapy fit well with all psychiatric diagnoses and therapies. One can assess organic illness and biologic factors, interpersonal psychodynamics, family interactions, and the family's relationship with society. General systems theory and the bio-psychosocial model of medical practice provide a broad frame of reference to which these diverse approaches to data gathering may be related. As there is not yet a precise formula to handle such data, clinical judgment must decide which elements are more important, but they all should be considered before any is discarded or relegated to a minor role.

When talking with a patient, the focus of the interview is, of necessity, on that person. I have pointed out the need to maintain a broad perspective so that relevant material is not missed. Nevertheless, one is accepting and should accept a view of the patient's world as he or she sees it.

When the doctor sits with a family in the doctor's office, hospital, or at the family's home, the perspective immediately changes. You are no longer hearing only the patient's interpretation of his or her social environment, but other possibly conflicting interpretations of the scene. In addition, the physician is making his or her own private interpretations, which may not necessarily agree with any given by family members.

Interviews with family members, friends, employers, and others are indicated whenever they would help to corroborate the patient's account of problems, whenever additional information is needed, and whenever disturbed interpersonal relationships might be a major cause of the patient's problems. Usually, but not always, family members can help to evaluate a delusional system or to give additional information about the patient's behavior and symptoms at present, prior to, and at the time of onset of the illness. In interviewing family members, one should always be aware that their perceptions are also colored by emotions and by their involvement with the patient.

To maintain your relationship with the patient, ask his or her permission to talk with a family member or interested other person and tell the patient that no confidential information will be given to that person. For example, one can say, "I'd like to talk with your wife, who came with you today. How do you feel about that?" Most patients will give permission. Then go on to say, "I want you to know that I won't tell her any of the things we talked about. They are confidential between us." If the patient has questions about any of this, it may be better to talk with the family member in their presence. Some psychiatrists will not see family members at all or only with the patient present; however, it is best to have access to information from all possible sources. With proper consideration, this can be done without disrupting the doctor–patient relationship.

Most family members will want to know what the doctor thinks about the patient's condition, and you should tell them something. In the interests of a positive doctor–patient interaction, tell the patient in advance what will be told to the family about his or her condition. Say as little as possible to the family until family interaction is better known. Family members can use diagnosis as a club over a patient's head. A good thing to say to the patient is something like, "When I talk with your wife, she will probably want to know what I think about your problem. Do you have any ideas about what I should tell her?" Surprisingly, the patient's ideas may well agree with those of the interviewer. If so, this will solve the problem.

If the patient and the interviewer disagree, this should be discussed and some mutual decision arrived at. Some patients are more in need of protection and cannot participate in such decisions. Here, doctors should tell their patients that they need care or to be in the hospital and that the doctor will tell this to the patients' relatives. Patients should be given the opportunity to discuss their feelings about this.

The basic principles of psychiatric interviewing already discussed also apply to interviewing a family member. Help the person feel at ease and give the person an opportunity to say what is on his or her mind. After helping to reduce tension, one way to begin is to say, "I've seen your husband and he agreed that it would be good for me to talk with you. Perhaps you could tell me how you see the situation." As with patient interviews, some people ask for more structure. If so, the doctor could respond by saying, "When did you first notice a change?" or "When did the problem begin?" Usually, you need only give the family member permission to talk.

Interviewing a patient and individual family members is not a family assessment. Family interviewing encompasses more variables. Family interviews are designed to gain an understanding of family dynamics and the family's interaction with society as these relate to the patient. As treatment progresses, some modification in the interactions adversely affecting the patient can be made. Family therapy may be undertaken by those with training in the field. I will only discuss here family interviewing for assessment.

It is "important to differentiate the process of family interviewing from that of family therapy. By separating one from the other, differing objectives can be conceptualized. Once having recognized that several family interviews are not the same thing as therapy of a family, clinicians become freer to use such interviews for planning appropriate clinical management without feeling constrained to do family therapy.

The result is increased clinical flexibility and a broader basis on which to make decisions about the modalities to be used. Moreover, when family interviews are introduced early, their intercurrent use during subsequent treatment feels natural and relatively uncomplicated" (Brown 1980).

A series of family diagnostic interviews can be therapeutic, as can a series of individual diagnostic interviews. Even so, the family interview should be viewed as a tool to help the patient and is thus differentiated from family therapy.

I have discussed the need for and ways of maintaining the relationship with the primary patient. When working with the patient and his or her family, maintaining this relationship may be more difficult, because we want to also impart a feeling of importance to each family member. Howells discusses the importance of the interviewer's relationship with the family. "Built into the formal investigatory procedure is every device for enriching the rapport with the family. The golden road to the elucidation of the intimate, significant and meaningful psychopathology is a sustained deep rapport between the investigators and the family. To follow with precision the procedure suggested could yield, on its own, virtually no useful information. Rapport brings the procedure to life. It is at this point, rapport, that the machine can fail; it requires a warm, tolerant, understanding human relationship to touch and encourage the hurt, embarrassed chords of memory to express themselves. Rapport makes for security, security for communication, and communication for meaningful information" (Howells 1975).

We will be trying to maintain rapport in a situation where several family members, or at least more than one, depending on the number being interviewed, will probably vie for special attention from the doctor. As long as the doctor is aware of this, like transference, it will give the doctor an opportunity to observe how family members' individual psychological problems show as they compete with each other for recognition. How does the patient handle this competition from other family members?

Sometimes family visits will take place at home, affording an opportunity to view the house and the surrounding neighborhood. Students completing clerkships or special programs in community mental health centers or neighborhood health programs will have an opportunity for family assessment in the home. However, most families will be seen when the patient is brought to the hospital or clinic or they will be asked to come specifically for a family interview.

The room used for a family interview should be comfortable and large enough, but not too large to get lost in. It should have a variety of seating arrangements such as a sofa and adequate number of chairs so as to permit options in the family seating arrangements. The family is invited into the room and, as they come in, the assessment begins.

Observation of nonverbal and verbal behavior as the family comes into the room is quite revealing. Facial expression, eye contact, manner of walk, social distance, all nonverbal behavior to be observed in a single patient are important in family units and are difficult to make. The interviewer is trying to observe several people and their interactions at almost the same time. Any conclusions drawn from these observations must be equally tentative; nevertheless, they will yield important data to be combined with that already obtained from the patient and more to be obtained later.

Seating preference of each family member is another clue to relationships. Is the patient isolated, are any other family members apparently excluded, or do any exclude themselves?

After everyone is seated, the interviewer should introduce himself or herself and ask each member of the family to introduce themselves. The presence of each family member should be acknowledged. The interviewer must then state the purpose of the interview to the entire family. A family interview, being a less familiar situation than an individual interview, will require more explanation. A patient usually knows why he or she is seeing the doctor and has at least a notion of what to expect. The family does not know exactly what to expect. Some family members may not even want to be there, or they may not want other members of the family to be there.

The family interview therefore requires more explanation from the interviewer. The interviewer can begin by saying that this is an opportunity to get to know the family, that this meeting had been discussed with the patient, who agreed that it would be a good idea. Or, if the patient agreed reluctantly, this can be stated so that the interview begins with openness and honesty. The interviewer can say that problems of family members usually have some effect on everyone and that others in the family might have things that they want to discuss. At this point, one could ask the parent or spouse, or whoever, how he or she felt about coming today. This might well open the discussion and lead to important areas. Or, one can ask if any of the family members know of problems that the patient might be reacting to. Other interviewers might start by asking, "How can I help you?" Just as with the individual interview, it is best to start with an open-ended question.

In an individual interview, one usually can safely let the expression of negative feelings run their course (unless the patient's hostility is about to get out of control). Indeed, it may be therapeutic to do so. In a family interview, such expression may be therapeutic, but the effect on others must be carefully monitored. Until one gains more experience, it is better to err on the side of conservatism and not let the discussion focus negatively on any one person for very long. The clinician should observe and allow the expression of negative feelings, but for a family interview to be successful, the situation cannot become intolerable for anyone. The interviewer treads a fine line between being a Pollyanna or conducting a bland interview, or allowing controlled expression of feelings. Because family interviews are more difficult, a second interviewer in the room may help to make additional observations or occasionally step in and help out.

The interviewer must, from time to time, support a member of the family as that person expresses his or her feelings and point of view; however, the doctor must not constantly take the side of any family member during the interview. It is more difficult to avoid this than it is to be objective about an individual patient. Families have alliances that outsiders are easily pulled into.

Everyone should have a chance to speak during the interview. The interviewer may have to turn directly to a person who has not talked at all and ask what he or she thinks about the subject under discussion, especially if the subject relates to that individual. A family interview requires much more active participation by the interviewer. This may mean interrupting a particularly talkative and dominant family member in order to allow a more passive one to participate. You may have to support actively a member under attack with a statement such as, "We are not here to make any judgments. What we want to do is see if there is any way that we can help." Such statements are made not in a critical but in a supportive manner.

As observations bring in more systems and get farther from the specific details being studied, the more general the theories become for relating these observations. So it is with a frame of reference used to understand the family system as it relates to the psychiatric patient and to society. A number of theories and interactional models are used to understand families, discussion of which is beyond the scope of this book. Here we will discuss a simpler way of making some sense out of the family interview for the benefit of the patient.

Using the mental status and psychiatric history for guidance, we can assess the family unit as a whole, make observations of individual members and their relationships, and learn something of important historical events in the family. This model can also be used to develop guidelines for recording the family interview. All items primarily developed for individuals will not apply to the family.

Observations about general appearance, behavior, and speech are made of the family unit and of the members in relation to each other. The focus is no longer only on a specific individual. Observations may be on an individual, but these are immediately interpreted in the context of the family unit and that person's relationship with others in the family. I have mentioned observing nonverbal behavior as the family enters the room and the possible meaning of the seating arrangements chosen. You should also note age, sex, dress, and personal appearance of family members. Any disparities are usually readily apparent, and include such things as marked differences in age between husband and wife or marked difference in personal appearance. As with observations made in the individual interview, put such disparities in the back of your mind as questions for possible future exploration.

Here are some observations made early in a family interview that was part of an evaluation of a four-year-old boy, who was referred because of hyperactivity and aggression:

> Jim was seen with his parents. The parents were casually, but neatly, dressed. Mrs. S is slender and reserved. Mr. S is of medium height, muscular, and quite verbal. He prevented his wife from saying much. He frequently indulged in overly detailed descriptions of problems that were not entirely relevant. Mrs. S did not seem inclined to present material or give her point of view even when given the opportunity. When she did talk, Mr. S would sometimes interrupt her to clarify a factual matter. Jim was well-developed for his age. He did not speak out, was very active and moved about the room from object to object. The father appeared to ignore him until he did something disruptive, but the mother followed his every move.

The family's manner of relating to the examiner and to each other is of special importance. I have discussed some aspects of this, such as attempts by one family member to get the examiner to side with another family member. The family interview also gives the examiner an opportuniity to note how the patient relates in the presence of his or her family. The examiner might be surprised that this relationship has an entirely different quality from the dyadic relationship of doctor and patient. Any differences are noteworthy.

With several people together, there are so many bits of behavior and so many interactions that it is difficult for observers to keep up with them. You should note many things that can be recorded later. For example, how does one family member behave when another is talking? The family may be relatively relaxed until a particular member—it might be the patient—begins to say something, then everyone tenses up. Or, one might see a look of boredom or disgust on the face of one family member while another is talking. As with individual interviews, until one knows the situation well, it is not a good idea to make explicit statements about these observations. However, it is often appropriate to turn to a member of the family who obviously has some feelings about what is being said and simply ask them their thoughts about the subject under discussion.

Sometimes the patient, or a relative, may become so upset during the course of the interview that he or she must leave the room. If one notes mounting tension, in the first interview say, "What we are discussing does seem to cause a lot of feelings—maybe more than people can handle right now, and it might be well to go on to something else and come back to this later, if necessary."

Families have their own particular moods that seem to prevail most of the time. There are depressed families, anxious families, and angry families, among others. Is the prevailing mood appropriate? Is the general mood appropriate to the interview situation? Coming in to talk to the doctor about an illness in a family member is serious and somewhat depressing. This is the general attitude one might expect the family to have. Marked deviation from this should be noted. As matters come up during the course of the interview, one can determine whether or not the affect is appropriate to them.

Sensorium and intellectual functioning are not directly tested in a family interview, but that does not mean that the interviewer should not make some observations about them. Again, it is important to note if there is a marked discrepancy in one family member as compared with the others. Are the intellectual functioning of husband and wife, for example, approximately the same, or is there a marked difference? If so, this might cause tension within the family. Rarely does one see someone who is completely disoriented in a family interview, but this does happen and certainly should be explored.

In making a rough assessment of family mental status, note the predominant themes discussed during the course of the interview. Especially important are preoccupations of the family and individual family members. Are the preoccupations appropriate, or are they about something unrelated to the problems at hand? What is the insight into the problem, and what judgments are being made about how to cope? To paraphrase Harry Stack Sullivan (1954), in gathering information about a family we want to know who is this family and how did they come to be here? Every family has a unique history, unique set of problems, and their own particular ways of trying to cope with these problems. Some ways of coping are successful, others are not.

The psychosocial history of the family can follow developmental lines as does an individual psychosocial history. We want to know something about the development of the family unit itself: meeting and courtship of the spouses, marriage, and the development of that marriage. Do not go into the birth and development of individual family members in as much detail as with the individual patient; obtain this information as it seems important. The interviewer wants to know something about the parents of a couple and something about the couple's early lives. This influences their relationships with each other, just as the early history of an individual is an important factor in his or her present life. All that I have said about the importance of early childhood history to an individual patient applies also to each member of a family and helps to determine the interactions within that family.

Finally, do not neglect the family's relationship to the larger society. You need to know the circumstances of their living: what sort of house, the neighborhood they live in, what groups the family relates to, and, especially, how they see themselves fitting into the community and the world at large.

It takes several hours to get a complete family history and a developmental history for each member of the family, but this is rarely necessary. The interviewer is interested in how the family sees the patient's illness. When and how did it begin and how has it progressed? What problems was the family having at the onset of the patient's problems? Are there earlier problems that may have contributed?

Some Special Areas to Observe in the Family System

When interviewing an individual, the interviewer attempts to set up circumstances so that the patient is free to say what is on his or her mind. With the family interview, one attempts to provide an atmosphere that allows family members to interact with one another.

The family is to be observed as an interactional system and not simply as individuals who happen to reside together. The interviewer will do whatever possible to allow some interaction among family members. You could conduct a family interview by talking with each relative individually, but this would not promote the family interaction. Rather, if members of the family want to have a discussion within the interview, this should be encouraged. Their comments about what other family members have said or what the interviewer has said are to be encouraged.

Lewis (1980) states, "To obtain data about the family system requires a procedure that promotes interaction among the family members. The clinician's observations would focus on the nature of the interaction, particularly on those repetitive exchanges that appear to be patterns."

Various books on family therapy characterize interactional patterns differently. According to Reiss (1980), one looks for an interplay of relationships, what is said and done, who does what to whom, and a temporal sequence of events. These usually quickly sort themselves into patterns that the clinician can observe.

I will briefly discuss some interactional patterns that can be observed. Other authors may describe some of these differently.

LEADERSHIP ROLES

Who occupies leadership in various areas and in what way is this leadership carried out? In a more healthy, stable family, leadership is shared. Even though specific areas in which parents exert leadership may be changing due to the changing roles of men and women in our culture, one parent will generally assume more leadership in one area, the other parent in another area; but important decisions are often shared.

Parents must provide leadership for young children. Without this, chaos may develop, or children will assume leadership prematurely and thus give up a certain amount of their freedom to develop in their own way. Sometimes parental leadership roles are markedly deviant from the society in which the family resides. If this is the case, it should be noted because it might present a problem.

COALITIONS

Coalitions of two or more family members against another or others in the family may occur. An interviewer can easily become caught up in these coalitions and inadvertently take sides. Unhealthy coalitions often develop in the family, especially certain parent–child coalitions against another parent or coalitions of all family members against a particular child.

DOMINANT–SUBMISSIVE RELATIONSHIPS

Dominant–submissive relationships are not difficult to observe in the family interview. One frequently sees one parent doing all the talking or one parent offering all the opinions over those of the other. A child may not be allowed to talk or may choose to be submissive.

PARENTAL-NURTURING FUNCTIONS

Parents must be able to take care of children and provide the atmosphere for them to grow. They must provide certain basic functions of protection: the necessities of life and decision-making in relation to the outside world. Mature parents are able to do this. Others may not be able to.

FAMILY COMPETENCE

Lewis and colleagues (1976) have developed a method of assessing family competence, based on assessment of a large number of variables in the family interactional system. Families can be divided into four groups: optimal families, competent but pained families, dysfunctional families, and severely dysfunctional families. The extremes in this continuum can be distinguished by gross observation. "For example, the optimal families were characterized by clear structure with flexibility, dysfunctional families by unclear but rigid structures, and severely dysfunctional families by unclear structure. Therefore, one continuum (overt power) ranges from flexibility to rigidity to chaos" (Lewis 1980).

In optimal families, the leadership role is shared but each parent is capable of providing leadership. There are no unhealthy coalitions and there are warm, satisfying relationships between and among family members.

Severely dysfunctional families are not able to support maturation and growth of children. The family may be chaotic, with no clearly defined person in a leadership role and no meaningful communication about decisions being made. These families have poor relationships with the outside world.

Family competence can be assessed in the areas of socioeconomic, personal, and interpersonal relationships. Evaluating family competence, and some of the more specific interactions that relate to it, is a major function of the family interview.

GENDER-LINKED ROLES

Male and female roles are defined by culture and society, and these, in turn, have an impact on how they are acted out within the family. The family interviewer can observe these roles and the ways in which parents help their children develop and identify.

PURSUIT OF INDIVIDUAL NEEDS VERSUS FAMILY NEEDS

Both personal and family needs are important. In competent, mature families both may be pursued: the needs of the family can be met, children's needs can be met by parents, and individuals can also pursue their own areas of interest and gain satisfaction from them.

As the family interview develops, you may find that the family's present problem is not the patient at all, but a serious family crisis to which the patient may be reacting. A short series of interviews may be indicated to help the family resolve the crisis. Langsley and Kaplan (1968) demonstrated that much could be accomplished by crisis intervention.

Family crises usually relate to a number of predictable things: major illness or death of a family member; change of residence; children leaving home; changes in economic status. Economic change can be in either direction: a loss of finances or a major promotion for one of the working members of the family which shakes the family's status quo significantly enough to necessitate adaptive changes in other members. Popular literature is now replete with crises brought on when women are given promotions or assume new roles in the working world. You may be surprised to learn that this is not a new problem. It has been occurring for generations, particularly in underdeveloped areas where industries employ women in textile weaving, garment making, and now electronics. In some of these areas, men who were farmers or laborers no longer have work and they must adjust to a different role in the family and in their society.

As with the individual, the medical history of the family can be taken. This is an abbreviated medical history of individuals and how these may affect the family as a whole.

Although I have been talking about family interviewing in relation to psychiatric patients, an understanding of the family is also important for the primary care physician. The term "family physician" may be somewhat of a misnomer if he or she is so designated because all members of the family, regardless of age, are treated. That does not necessarily mean that he or she treats the family as a unit and, indeed, many family physicians do not. Yet, this is important not only for the total health of the family but also with such specific problems as compliance with prescribed medical regimes. A patient is more apt to take medication properly if he or she has the support and understanding of the family. Even if the medication is taken, the effects on the patient's well-being may very well be influenced by the family situation and attitudes.

Family Assessment

The P family assessment was made by several groups of medical students, who were asked to make a home visit because Mrs. P was not bringing her children to the clinic at the proper time for their immunizations. When she did come, she was distraught and quick to anger. This family report illustrates many areas relevant in a family assessment and also shows family changes through time.

INITIAL VISIT: FEBRUARY

Mrs. P is the mother of four children and is in good health. The household consists of six members, five living in the house:

Mr. P, 31 years of age and not living in the house

Mrs. P, 27 years of age

Mary, 4½ years of age

Harold, 3½ years of age

Frank, 2½ years of age

Martha, 1 year of age

The family lives in a three-room, one-bath, wood-frame duplex. Mrs. P's sister and her family live in the other half of the duplex. After a recent robbery, they built a doorway between the apartments to help Mrs. P feel more secure.

The family has a kitchen, bedroom, and combination living room/ bedroom. The house needs paint and repair: the steps are rotten and the door has holes in it. A latch on the fence is broken and there is a junked car in the driveway. There are some flowers planted in the front yard. The grass needs cutting. The clothesline is full of washed clothes. The furnishings are in good condition, but the refrigerator works only occasionally.

Mrs. P depends entirely on a monthly welfare check. Out of this, comes rent, an undetermined amount for utilities, and money for food stamps. Mrs. P does not work now because of her children and the loss of welfare payments if she did work. She would like to work in the future. She was a maid at a motel before her marriage. As a child she helped her family, who were migrant farm workers. As a result of moving from place to place, she completed only the sixth grade.

Mrs. P manages her money well. She preplans what bills to pay and knows how much money might be left, which she spends for children's clothes or on necessities such as toilet paper and laundry soap. She cuts corners by giving her children haircuts and making some of their clothes. Sometimes she splurges on something for the children, but not often. She does not buy beyond her means and has bought only once on credit: a television, on which she still owes money. Mrs. P admits her biggest problem is money, but she does not see the situation as hopeless. As soon as she is able she wants to work to earn money for her family, most of all for her children's schooling.

Mrs. P cares about her home and works hard to make it look good. She has plastered the holes in the walls and cleaned the exterior. She plans to fix the pipes and repair the damage caused by vandals. Unfortunately, she must pay for all of this herself and it will take a long time. More depressing than the thought of the money is that if the house looks too good it will be robbed again. The vandals stole her new television (unpaid for), her mother's sewing machine, most of her clothes and linens, her food staples, and destroyed what they could not take. The neighborhood is bad, compounding her poverty with fear.

Mrs. P states that she was deserted by her husband, who returned to Mexico.

SOCIAL HISTORY

Mrs. P was born and reared in a city in the Southwest, where she and her family have lived all their lives. They have lived at their present address for approximately five months. Before that they lived in squalor for five years at another place. The house had no indoor bathroom, no running water, no hot water, and was infested with rats and roaches. Mrs. P's husband deserted the family there.

Mrs. P's father is dead, and her mother lives close by. She has nine brothers and nine sisters, all but one of whom are married. Mrs. P has a grandmother, who is in her 80s. Her mother completed the fifth grade and her father the third grade. All family members were migrant farm workers.

Mrs. P resents her father because he was strict and severe. He would not allow the children to have friends or toys. He would not allow Mrs. P to help her mother in the kitchen and, therefore, she knew nothing about household chores when she married. She is trying hard not to make her children suffer as she did.

Mrs. P was 22 years old when she married Jim P, whom she met while working at the motel; he was there on a work permit from Mexico. They knew each other for six months before they were married. According to Mrs. P, this was a "big mistake." Because her father isolated her so much, Jim was the first man she had ever known. She jumped into marriage "to get away from my father and the emptiness." There were many problems. He spoke only Spanish and, therefore, she had to go with him as a translator when he was job hunting, shopping, and so on. This made it impossible for her to get any work done, much less raise a family. Moreover, he would not allow English to be spoken at home and became violent when she did not obey. He stayed out nights and drank excessively. She feared for herself and her children. Finally, he deserted her and went to Mexico for a divorce. She is hurt and bitter about her marriage and says she "will never marry again."

She is going to devote her life to her children. She wants an education for them so they can get good jobs and work for a living. She will do anything for them. They appear to realize this and work with her, helping in every way possible. The children seem self-sufficient for their ages. The oldest helps care for the youngest. Mrs. P's chief concern is the care, health, and schooling of her family. She makes her home the center of everything. She watches television with her children, teaches them, and sometimes takes them to the park. When she goes out, the entire family goes out. Everything is shared.

Mrs. P appears to be isolated from the rest of the world, trusting only her family to help her, and fearing everyone and everything else. She does not know any of her neighbors and will not make an attempt to know them.

She attends church regularly with her mother; her children also attend. The oldest attends preschool and is progressing well academically and socially. Her school activities have drawn her mother out of the house. Mrs. P is now considering several craft programs, such as knitting and sewing. She has taken her children to the clinic for examinations and plans to take advantage of the public assistance dental care plan. All her dealings with the health institutions have been good.

MARCH

Before the next interview with the family, Mr. P, the presumed former husband, returned. This complicated the assessment of the family. There were major discrepancies between what Mrs. P had said and the information obtained from Mr. P.

He related that he did not drink and was a mild-mannered person who always remained calm. According to him, he filed for a divorce because he could not find a job. If he was not living at home and had divorced his wife, she would be eligible for welfare and would at least have a regular income. Also, he said he left the family to go to Mexico, where he was hoping to find a job, earn some money, and send for his family at a later date. Like his wife, he expressed a deep love and affection for his children, which showed in both actions and words. He often spoke of the need for them to have an education and how he loved them and wanted to be with them. During the interview, he held his oldest daughter close to him and would rustle one of his sons' hair.

Mrs. P seems to remind her husband constantly that he is in the United States only because he married her, that he cannot speak English and therefore cannot get a job, and that she might have to work to support her family.

APRIL

When we arrived at the P home, we found the family enjoying a relaxing afternoon. Mrs. P was in the backyard spraying water on the children with a garden hose. In the living room Mr. P sat with his sister-in-law, who was teaching him how to crochet. He appeared to be enjoying himself. Mrs. P came in to greet us.

Mr. P had not yet found a job, although he stated that he had made another application since the last time we had seen him. He did not seem too concerned that he had not found a job (in contrast to previous occasions when he seemed very anxious and worried). Mr. P continued his crocheting. Mrs. P mentioned that she was still babysitting and that the food stamp office would not approve their application until she delivers a paper certifying how much she earns per week. She also informed me that their car's transmission "went on the blink" the previous week. Otherwise, everything was the same and everyone was doing well.

MAY

I spoke with Mrs. P at the door for only a few minutes. She claimed to be ill and immediately asked that I return another day. She seemed to have just woken up; the house was closed up tight and the living room was messy and unorganized. She told me that her husband had found employment as a gardener for the city.

SEPTEMBER

Mr. P is holding a steady job as a gardener for the city parks service. Both he and his wife continue to care for the children well, but Mr. P is more openly expressive than Mrs. P of his affection for them. He more frequently romps and plays with the children. Mrs. P thinks this spoils them, and he is therefore given less responsibility in disciplining the children.

SUMMER, THE FOLLOWING YEAR

Two of the boys were standing on the porch as we walked up to the house. Mrs. P greeted us warmly after we had knocked on the door. Her hair was combed; she was wearing clean shorts and top and flowered tennis shoes without laces.

The inside of the house was clean. The furniture was neatly arranged and the floor looked recently swept. The furnishings were a mixture of old and new: the sofa we sat on was torn; we could see that the refrigerator in the kitchen was a new model. She had a fancy mixer and can opener. The television was on throughout the interview.

One of the most important events that occurred in the family was Mrs. P's obtaining a job. She explained that Mr. P's salary was not enough to pay the bills, so she had to get a job. The problem became acute when their television was stolen. They were told that, even though it was stolen, they still had to pay for it. Mrs. P at first refused; however, the company threatened to take her to court, so she is now paying monthly for the television. She had found a job as a motel maid. For the most part, she was satisfied with the job.

Along with her job, she incurred extra expenses. She must pay for a live-in maid who takes care of the children five days a week while Mr. P takes care of them on weekends. She must also pay a neighbor to take her to work. She does not have any regular days off: her boss tells her each week when her days off will be. The financial problem is compounded because they now receive no food stamps or other aid. Mrs. P explained that when she got her new job, the welfare office wanted to know how much she made, but, since her schedule was irregular, she could not tell them. Now she knows her salary; however, she has been unable to return to the welfare office to reapply for food stamps.

Mrs. P said that despite the fact that both she and her husband have to work, they still manage to go dancing or to the movies once in a while. The P family seems to have coped with some of their problems. One of these is their financial problem. They were behind in one of their bills, so Mrs. P decided she had to get a job.

References

Brown SL: Family interviewing as a basis for clinical management, in Hofling CK, Lewis JM (eds): *The Family: Evaluation and Treatment*. New York, Brunner/Mazel, 1980.

Howells JG: *Principles of Family Interviewing*. New York, Brunner/Mazel, 1975.

Langsley DG, Kaplan DM: *The Treatment of Families in Crisis*. New York, Grune & Stratton, 1968.

Lewis JM: The family matrix in health and disease, in Hofling CK, Lewis JM (eds): *The Family: Evaluation and Treatment*. New York, Brunner/Mazel, 1980.

Lewis JM, Beavers WR, Gossett JT, Phillips VA: *No Single Thread: Psychological Health in Family Systems*. New York, Brunner/Mazel, 1976.

Reiss D: Pathways to assessing the family: some choice points and a sample route, in Hofling CK, Lewis JM (eds): *The Family: Evaluation and Treatment*. New York, Brunner/Mazel, 1980.

Sullivan HS: *The Psychiatric Interview*, Perry HS, Gawel ML (eds). New York, Norton, 1954.

11

The Family Physician and the Psychiatric Interview

James M. Turnbull, MD, FRCP(C)

A significant proportion of mental health care in the United States is provided to nonhospitalized patients by physicians who are not psychiatrists (Schurman et al 1985a, 1985b). For this reason, most family practice residency programs place considerable emphasis on the acquisition of knowledge in the discipline of psychiatry. Interviewing skills are usually taught during the first year of most residency programs. Despite this emphasis, the average family practitioner does not conduct a well-disciplined, purposeful diagnostic and therapeutic psychiatric interview. The reasons for this are fourfold: time, focus, interest level, and attitude.

Time

Most family doctors feel under the pressure of time during the majority of their working day. They are constantly interrupted by the telephone, experience the stress of a waiting room full of patients, frequently fall behind (and are therefore late for appointments), and have the added imposition of "walk-ins" (patients who come without an appointment). They are also frustrated by arguments with insurance carriers about recertification and the necessity for patients to be hospitalized. Thus, they see the psychiatric patient who presents with a new symptom as an intrusion on the hallowed 15 minutes allotted most patients. The race with time, like most other dimensions of life that we attempt to control, is very much a chimera. When properly used, time works to the advantage of the family physician. It is relatively easy to establish the discipline of refusing to be interrupted by the telephone except during certain periods of the day and to return telephone calls to patients or to pharmacies at preset times. Family physicians can train their receptionists and their nurse to allow them to maximize their own time and also to screen patients who may require more time than others.

The physician who presents to his or her patients the attitude of "always being on the run" can rarely establish the degree of rapport necessary to be helpful when a psychiatric symptom occurs. Most patients who present with psychiatric symptoms can be rescheduled for further interviewing when the physician feels under less pressure. This may require advance planning so that the patients are not frustrated when the appointment secretary informs them that the doctor has no openings available for several weeks. Sometimes the physician feels that patients should instinctively know how busy he or she is. For the patient, however, the time spent with his or her doctor is of much greater importance than the physician's busy schedule.

Focus

Most family physicians are interested in obtaining an accurate diagnosis as rapidly and with as little cost to the patient as possible. The diagnostic process is sometimes seen as an essential hurdle before the physician's real skill, treatment, is brought into play. Speed, then, is of the essence. The physician may launch into an immediate interrogative style, wishing to complete a review of systems as rapidly as possible and allowing listening skills so essential to the psychiatric interview to take a very secondary place. Being able to focus requires being able to shift mental gears. For most psychiatric patients, the focus needs to be redirected. The physician needs to be a more active listener and to ask fewer questions. Interrogative interviewing frequently indicates that the interviewer is anxious, and anxiety notoriously interferes with one's ability to listen accurately. The interviewer needs to change his or her focus from active intervener to reflective thinker.

Interest Level

A great deal has been written about the subtle psychopathology seen in its many guises in the family physician's office. The interest level of family physicians for psychiatric illness varies considerably from individual to individual. Although much lip service is given to the importance of training in psychiatry, many family doctors think its importance is overrated and tend to lose interest when patients present with psychiatric symptoms. Many family physicians have the mistaken attitude that psychiatric illness is incurable and always long-term. These attitudes toward psychiatry are unfortunate because they tend to diminish the amount of interest displayed in the discipline by the average family physician.

Attitude

Attitudes towards psychiatry are often entrenched in the potential family physicians even before they attend medical school. Many family doctors see the psychiatrist, and by extension psychiatric patients, as being out of the general domain of medicine and not relevant to their own particular practice. Although family doctors are supposed to have some understanding of family dynamics, they frequently fail to understand how these affect the illness of family members. Changes in attitude towards psychiatric patients can come about only by positive experiences both with psychiatrists and with patients with psychiatric symptoms.

Use of Time

PATIENT: Thank you for fitting me in, doctor. I have been feeling really lousy lately, you know, kind of nervous all the time.

FAMILY DOCTOR: Tell me more about how you have been feeling.

PATIENT: Well, I guess it's just nerves. I get these feelings like I am going to faint, like I may throw up. It's really bad when I get home at night after work.

FAMILY DOCTOR: When you get home?

PATIENT: Yes, my wife and I haven't been getting along too well lately.

It now becomes apparent that this interview will need to be continued later. The physician does not now have the time to take an extended history of the current situation.

FAMILY DOCTOR: Is this something recent?

PATIENT: Well, not exactly. It's been coming on for some time.

FAMILY DOCTOR: Do you think it would be a good idea if we set aside some time later this week to discuss this thoroughly?

PATIENT: I guess so, Doc. Maybe you could see my wife, too.

The essential elements of the psychiatric interview have been discussed in detail in other parts of this book. These are the same for the family physician as for any other physician, with certain special perspectives.

The family physician usually has less time to develop rapport with the patient than specialists in other fields. Because of the constraints already mentioned, particularly of time and focus, the physician must develop rapport within a very brief interview. He or she must be able to convey a feeling of compassion, understanding, and respect for the patient.

The revealing study by Korsch and Negrete (1972), which involved the careful review of doctor–patient encounters in a pediatric clinic, documented that a majority of the mothers were unhappy because the physician paid too little attention to their concern and apprehension about the child. When the videotapes of the interviews were reviewed later, the physician spoke more than the patient's parent 95 percent of the time. These tapes also revealed that 5 percent of the conversation with the parent had been friendly or personal in nature. Several other studies have shown that the characteristics of the encounter between the physician and the patient correlates highly with both patient and physician satisfaction (Starfield et al 1981; Weinberg et al 1981; Comstock et al 1982).

Family physicians should pay particular attention to body language and to other nonverbal cues. The majority of human expression is generated in the face, and physicians who spend much of the early part of the interview observing and collating data on the patient's amount of eye contact, general expression, the presence or absence of tearing, and observation of the five basic emotions (fear, anger, joy, sadness, and disgust) will have added considerably to their knowledge of what is going on with the patient. Of equal importance is knowledge of canceled appointments, missed appointments, and patients who have arrived late. This often relates to fear concerning the implications of both symptoms and treatment. This type of behavior requires early identification if rapport is to be enhanced and compliance obtained. Other patients will always come to the office accompanied by relatives or friends. This may indicate imagined seriousness assigned to the problem by the family, a method of negotiating family disagreement, or frank agoraphobia.

An important part of the development of the good family physician is the acquisition of listening skills. Many family physicians assume that from years of sitting in class listening to lectures they have acquired good listening skills and are surprised by the statement that listening is an active rather than a passive procedure. All this exposure to other people's voices sometimes seems to release a pent-up torrent of words, which are released over the productive years of the physician's life. Listening to the patient requires an expression of interest and concern, as shown by the attentive stance of the physician sitting forward in the chair, looking interested, with his or her head slightly tilted. Family physicians who remain standing rather than sitting convey to the patients that they are in a hurry and wish to be somewhere else. Paul Fink (1987), the president of the American Psychiatric Association, when asked by a family physician what one piece of advice he would give to doctors to increase rapport with patients stated, "Sit down." Some family physicians only feel comfortable visiting patients at the hospital or in an examining room when the patient is horizontal and the physician is vertical. Other physicians will sit straddled over the chair with arms over the back of the chair, a defensive posture that makes good listening very difficult.

A simple exercise to help the family physician develop good listening skills is to spend two days in the office asking no direct questions of any patients. Instead the physician adopts an indirect style using statements like, "Tell me about . . . ," or "Describe for me as accurately as you can . . . ." This concentrates the skills in acquiring information without the use of direct questions and leads to much greater attention to the answers, changes, and speech patterns of the patient as well as to the information being conveyed. It is sometimes difficult for the family physician to allow the patient to stray off the point. Similarly, he or she feels anxious when there are periods of silence, being again frustrated by that omnipresent element of "time."

Finally, the ability to close an interview is something that most family physicians struggle over with patients who have psychiatric complaints. They sometimes believe that the interview process is neverending and are reluctant to draw the interview to a close when they are not sure they have covered everything. The technique of closing an interview after sufficient time has elapsed is a skill that has to be learned. The brief psychiatric interview, as practiced by most family physicians, has to recognize the importance of preparing the patient for ending. This should be done three or four minutes before the interview is concluded with a statement such as, "You have given me a great deal of helpful information today. I wonder if, before we close, there is any other important issue we need to deal with in the remaining few minutes?" Often the movement from one chair in an office to the chair behind the desk or reaching for a prescription pad is a helpful sign to the patient that the interview is about to end.

Communication skills are best taught and learned by the family doctor in a nonthreatening environment with a good role-modeling teacher. One program, developed at McMaster University, found that 87 percent of 110 residents could learn the necessary skills to assess and treat psychological symptoms in patients in such a setting (Lesser 1981). The family physician who wishes to improve his or her interviewing technique should practice establishing rapid rapport, observing body language, attending to other nonverbal cues, acquiring good listening skills, and learning how to close the interview. It is a relatively easy task, with practice, to use the skills delineated here in the brief time the physician has available in his or her office.

References

Comstock LM, Hooper EM, Goodwin JM, Goodwin JS: Physician behaviors that correlate with patient satisfaction. *J Med Educ* 1982;57:102–112.

Fink P: From a speech made at the meeting of the American Association of Social Psychiatry, New Orleans, Sept 1987.

Korsch BM, Negrete V: Doctor/patient communication. *Sci Am* 1972;227:66–74.

Lesser AL: The psychiatrist and family medicine: a different training approach. *Med Educ* 1981;15:398–406.

Schurman RA, Kramer PD, Mitchell JB: The hidden mental health network: treatment of mental illness by nonpsychiatrist physicians. *Arch Gen Psychiatry* 1985;42:89–94.

Schurman RA, Mitchell JB, Kramer PD: When doctors listen: counseling patterns of nonpsychiatrist physicians. *Am J Psychiatry* 1985;142:934–938.

Starfield B, Wray C, Hess K, Gross R, Birk PS, D'Lugoff BC: The influence of patient–practitioner agreement on outcome of care. *Am J Public Health* 1981;71:127–131.

Weinberg M, Greene JY, Mamlin JJ: The impact of clinical encounter events on patient and physician satisfaction. *Soc Sci Med* 1981;15e:239–244.

12

Interviewing the Patient with a Sexual Problem
James M. Turnbull, MD, FRCP(C)

In discussions with family physicians at meetings in many states, the statement has often been made to me, "I know that sex is important, but I never seem to get around to asking about it!" There are at least four reasons why primary care physicians fail to elicit data about the sexuality of their patients. These are:

Fear of embarrassing the patient

Anxiety on the part of the physician about the data being elicited

A failure to recognize the importance of a sexual history

Lack of a knowledge base on which to build a treatment strategy

Masters and Johnson have repeatedly commented in public that 50 percent of all adults in the United States have a sexual problem at some time in their lives sufficiently severe to warrant intervention. The person from whom most of these patients seek advice is their primary care doctor.

There are two types of sexual history: the screening history and the problem-oriented history (Munjack and Oziel 1980). The screening history is used to gather general data about sexual functioning in order to enhance overall diagnostic investigation and to provide education for the patient. The mnemonic E.L.I.C.I.T. summarizes the purposes of such a screening history.

E. Establishing the ambience of a setting in which the patient feels comfortable in discussing sexual concerns is very important. Sex is very private data. Patients are unlikely to reveal such personal material unless the physician shows concerns about the location in which the interview occurs and practices privacy. One patient of mine reported being asked about her sexual relationship while the physician had his door open, and the secretary outside the office immediately stopped typing.

L.I. This stands for limited information. Even in this day of "sexual enlightenment," many patients still believe myths acquired in early childhood and have many misconceptions about sexual functioning. Poor communication between partners about the nature of their sexual relationship is very common. One woman who was a patient of mine was turned off by the fact that her husband almost always drank before they attempted sexual intercourse. Yet she felt it would hurt his feelings too much to tell him that she would prefer him not to drink at this particular time.

C. The collection of data not only enables the physician to obtain important diagnostic clues, but also to determine whether the patient should be treated by him or her or referred. There are many illnesses in which a change in sexual performance is an early symptom (e.g., major depression, diabetes, multiple sclerosis). Sexual problems may also be side effects of a number of medications used in general medical practice. Of particular importance are depressants of the central nervous system and drugs used to treat hypertension.

I.T. Intensive therapy may be necessary for patients who are sexually dysfunctional. For most primary care physicians this will require a referral to someone who has more experience in treating sexual dysfunction, but there is no reason that family physicians should not be able to learn the necessary skills in order to treat such disorders in their own office.

The Screening History

INTRODUCTION

A good preliminary screening question is, "Are you generally satisfied with your sexual relationship?" This can be followed up with, "Is there anything about your sexual relationship you would like to see change?" Sometimes patients will respond to these questions as if there were no difficulties but will later return to the subject when they have had time to accept the information that the physician feels their sexual relationship is a topic of importance. I have had patients who six months after I had asked the preliminary question say, "You remember some time ago you asked me a question about my sexual relationship. Well, I didn't feel that I knew you well enough to talk to you about it at that time, but there are several difficulties."

When patients acknowledge the existence of a sexual dysfunction, the screening history then should determine the date of onset; the nature of the relationship and how much discordance exists; and whether treatment has been sought for the difficulties before. Indirect interviewing in order to obtain a sexual history is generally preferable to interrogation. Interrogative questions frequently reflect the interviewer's anxiety and tend to force the patient into a defensive posture. Areas of particular concern during the screening history include who initiates sexual advances, what variations in sexual activity occur, if any, myths and lack of information, as well as frequency or timing of sexual relations.

Many couples have difficulty in coming to some agreement as to how often they would like to share sexual activity. A statement to this effect may be helpful to a patient to express his or her concern. For example, the interviewer might say, "One of the most common problems patients have adjusting to one another has been how often they want sexual involvement. I wonder if that has been a problem for you?" One of the arenas for rejection in personal interaction is when making sexual overtures. Sometimes one or both partners avoid being the one to make advances because they are afraid the other will say, "No." It is amazing how quickly this can be cleared up when the primary care physician inquires about this particular aspect of the relationship with both members of the couple present.

Many medical conditions limit the patient's ability to engage in sexual expression, but these are more often produced psychologically than they are by physical constraints. Physicians who inquire about sexual functioning and reassure patients do a great service. This is particularly true in patients who have suffered mutilating surgery (e.g., breast surgery, or bowel surgery that results in a colostomy). Patients who have suffered myocardial infarction frequently need reassurance about reengaging in sexual activity following their hospitalization (Hellerstein and Friedman 1970).

MYTHS

In my experience, a number of men and women have acquired a lot of incorrect information about what happens to them as they age. Some women fear that they will undergo a significant loss of libido at the time of the menopause. Some men, who have experienced their first episode of erectile dysfunction, may fear that they are now totally impotent. Other myths are common and require education if they are to be corrected.

The Problem-Oriented History

The problem-oriented history develops naturally from the screening history. It has a number of purposes. First, this approach frequently helps differentiate between organically and psychologically based sexual dysfunction. Second, it clarifies the complexity of the problem and helps the physician decide whether to refer or to treat this patient himself. Third, and perhaps most important, it gives the physician insight into the way in which the couple communicate and conduct their interaction. The problem-oriented history poses a problem for most busy practitioners because of the time involved. For this reason, most physicians use one of the problem-oriented history forms that patients can take home with them. A number of these are available and have been devised by such experts in the field as LoPiccolo and LoPiccolo (1978), Masters and Johnson (1970), and Munjack and Oziel (1980). If one gives a patient a diagnostic questionnaire to take home, it is imperative that it be read by the treating physician when the patient returns for follow-up. Problem-oriented histories focus on a wide variety of areas. These include:

Childhood sexual experiences

The parental marriage and relationship

Early experience with sexual intercourse

The nature of the current sexual relationship

Common anxieties including initiation of sexual overtures, masturbation, fantasies, less than conventional forms of sexual expression

Extramarital affairs

Communication between partners about sexual matters

One exercise I have found useful for patients is to ask them to write three things they find attractive and helpful about their partners and three things they find unhelpful and destructive of the relationship. These are then read in the presence of both partners at the next interview.

When the problem-oriented history has been completed for both partners and the questionnaires have been studied, the formal process of taking the sexual history ends. At this time the primary care physician needs to make a decision about whether to treat the patients himself or to refer them.

References

Hellerstein HK, Friedman EH: Sexual activity of the post-coronary patient. *Arch Intern Med* 1970;125:987–999.

LoPiccolo J, LoPiccolo L (eds): *Handbook of Sex Therapy*. New York, Plenum, 1978.

Masters W, Johnson V: *Human Sexual Inadequacy*. Boston, Little Brown, 1970.

Munjack DJ, Oziel JL: *Sexual Medicine and Counseling in Office Practice*. Boston, Little Brown, 1980.

13

Elements of Psychotherapy

I have spoken often of the therapeutic value of the doctor–patient relationship. The development of rapport is essential for satisfactory progress in the interview. Because I strongly believe that any doctor–patient encounter can be therapeutic for the patient, I am including this chapter on the basic elements of psychotherapy. A knowledge of the theory of psychotherapy will help the reader to understand more about some of the procedures recommended in this book and to understand why we say that evaluation interviews have potential therapeutic value.

In contrast to the rest of this book, which tells how to interview psychiatric patients, this chapter does not tell how to conduct psychotherapy. There are many kinds of psychotherapies, and special training is required to master any one of them. Mastering the principles of interviewing presented in this book does give one a headstart toward learning psychotherapy. I will present here some basic principles that are common to many, if not all, psychotherapies. Although there are many psychotherapies, the theory presented is primarily that of psychoanalytically oriented psychotherapy.

Healing by psychological means is perhaps the most ancient of all healing methods. Although medicine men had a few specific plants and herbs with pharmacologically active ingredients, most of their therapeutic value was in the faith the patient had in the healer. Modern psychotherapy has attempted scientifically to develop psychological healing methods for patients who have mental problems resulting primarily from psychological causes. Because psychotherapy can help a patient improve his or her state of mind, it can indirectly benefit the patient's ability to deal with social and environmental problems. Furthermore, as studies have shown, psychotherapy improves patients' response to all treatment.

Because healing by psychological means is an ancient art, there are many old and new psychotherapies and many old and new theories about why they work. In recent years, we have seen a proliferation of psychotherapies. These range from simple counseling by well-meaning, but untrained, people, to elaborate rituals propounded by charlatans who may eventually turn a so-called therapy technique into a religion. Recent methods also include nude group therapy; feeling, touching, and pounding groups; primal scream therapy; and a host of others. Those promulgated by the more charismatic leaders are touted as new and miraculously effective.

Some therapies are stated to be effective because they expose primitive emotions. Others, such as rational therapy, are based on cognitive rather than emotional change. Many, such as transactional analysis, are aimed at both rational and emotional functions.

All these therapies have at least some basis for their claims even if they are often exploited by those who espouse them and may, in the wrong hands, be potentially harmful. Charismatic therapists may wittingly or unwittingly exploit the patient's trust or may in other ways stimulate more strongly the emotions causing the patient's trouble, making the patient worse, not better.

In psychoanalytically oriented psychotherapy, emotions already present are allowed to emerge in a controlled manner. The analyst does not provoke these feelings.

The mechanisms by which psychotherapy works are best understood at the psychological and behavioral level. Something must also happen at a biochemical and physiological level within the brain, otherwise psychotherapy would not be such an important concomitant therapeutic factor in many psychosomatic illnesses such as asthma, peptic ulcer, and others.

All psychotherapies have in common a therapist–patient relationship. This relationship must be trusting and hopeful for the patient, and the doctor should be empathic and accepting. The patient becomes somewhat dependent on the doctor, confident that the doctor has the patient's best interest in mind.

Frank (1975) says that within the context of this relationship the doctor has three aims: "The first is to enable the patient to discover new information about himself, both cognitively and experientially; the second is to arouse him emotionally, since emotions supply the emotive power for change; and the third is to encourage him to change his behavior in the light of what he has learned and to practice the new patterns."

Various schools of therapy give different emphasis to each of these areas. For example, existential therapy relies much more heavily on the power of the doctor–patient relationship to free the patient to experience present and future. Psychoanalysis leans heavily on the analysis of old patterns and feelings from the past as they are recreated in the doctor–patient relationship. Behavioral therapists place greater value on learning and practicing new behaviors.

In the first chapter I spoke at length about the doctor–patient relationship. All psychotherapies depend on the quality of that relationship. Some of its qualities are real and emanate from the personality and reputation of the therapist. Some depend on the perceptions of the patient and therapist. Both endow the relationship with emotional tones stemming from past relationships. In the patient this is called "transference," and in the therapist it is called "countertransference." The therapist must recognize his or her own countertransference so that it will not interfere with therapy. Dealing with the patient's transference reactions to the therapist is an important part of therapy.

The patient comes to the doctor needing help. The doctor provides a warm, empathic relationship and specific intervention when indicated. In this situation, the patient regresses and emotions from earlier life begin to emerge both directly and indirectly. Many of these emotions seem to the patient to somehow be stimulated by the therapist—this is the transference.

The same accepting, empathic relationship that allows the regression also provides an atmosphere in which both patient and therapist may look at and analyze irrational feelings and thoughts and the impact of these on the patient's present life. The therapist and patient form a therapeutic alliance in which, together, they analyze thoughts, feelings, and behavior that the patient finds troublesome. As a corollary to this therapeutic alliance, the patient develops a curious split in his or her personality. This is not pathological, but rather a healthy split that permits therapy to proceed.

This therapeutic split allows the patient to experience and express unacceptable thoughts and feelings and, at the same time, align the more mature part of his or her personality with the analytic functions of the therapist in order to observe and evaluate. What is immature and emerges from the past as a result of the dependency is simultaneously evaluated and put in rational, present-day perspective by therapist and patient working together. In this way, the patient is emotionally aroused and discovers new things about himself or herself.

As the process proceeds, patients find feelings and thoughts of which they were previously unaware. They learn more about themselves. Much of what they learn is from earlier times when they did not have adult strengths and resources to cope with problems. As these childhood conflicts are evaluated by the adult patient, they are seen differently and are no longer so formidable.

This rational look at old problems is not all that occurs in therapy.

The patient reexperiences the troublesome thoughts and feelings in a new relationship, with a new, if temporary, parent figure: the therapist. This has been called a corrective emotional experience. It is not a cognitive experience. Indeed, the patient may not even be able to put it into words. The patient feels differently because, as the old feelings emerge, the therapist acts differently from the parent. The patient feels accepted and no longer must fear retaliation for what is unacceptable.

This corrective emotional experience or experiential learning is a crucial factor in successful therapy. I have said before that the only insights valuable to a patient are his or her own insights. It is of little value for the doctor to tell patients the causes of their problems even if the doctor knows. This would be an intellectual insight, whereas the main problems are in the emotions. These must emerge and be experienced both emotionally and intellectually in the context of a new relationship.

Alexander and French (1946) describe the experience in this way: "In all forms of etiological psychotherapy, the basic therapeutic principle is the same: to reexpose the patient, under more favorable circumstances, to emotional situations which he could not handle in the past."

If all that I have so far described took place in a therapeutic situation, it would be helpful—the patient might feel better—but it would not be enough to effect the most desired results. As a final step, the patient must be willing and able to try new behavior, make mistakes if necessary, and learn from these efforts. Many an excellent therapeutic experience has faltered because a patient has not been able to take that additional step. If the patient can try new behavior, he or she finds new satisfactions and is more willing to discard old maladaptive patterns.

What has been presented is a simplified version of a complex process. Psychotherapy does not proceed so neatly nor always in the sequence outlined. For example, trying new behaviors may be followed by more regression during which hitherto unknown conflicts emerge. This is also not the psychotherapy for every patient or the choice of every psychiatrist. I have described without technical language a psychoanalytically oriented psychotherapy. It is a dynamic psychotherapy which presupposes that past emotional experience is a major determinant of present behavior.

Past emotional experience is not, however, the only determinant of present behavior. Heredity, physical health, cognitive learning, and the realities of the environment also play a part. No one immediately begins psychotherapy for an anxiety attack. The anxiety could be due to hyperthyroidism, panic disorder, or muggers in the neighborhood.

The psychiatric interview must assess all of these things so that correct intervention may be determined.

If physical and environmental factors are found to be of lesser importance and the patient appears motivated to understand himself or herself and try a new approach to some of his or her life situations, then most psychiatrists will begin psychoanalytically oriented psychotherapy. A significant number of psychiatrists, however, would choose behavior therapy. This therapy bypasses or puts less emphasis on understanding emerging feelings and thoughts. Its thrust is the development of specifically designed procedures to teach the patient new patterns of behavior.

As I have said, psychotherapy is a complex procedure requiring much skill and knowledge, which is acquired only after many years of training and experience. The learning and practice of psychotherapy is not suited to everyone: So is there something that physicians who are not psychiatrists can do to help their patients who want to discuss psychological and social problems as well as medical problems? Indeed there is, as we have commented throughout this book. We have also cited studies that show that patients may receive much help from a single interview.

All of the methods and techniques discussed will be helpful in what we call supportive psychotherapy (Karasu 1984). The doctor can first of all allow patients to talk, then listen and accept what they say. It can be helpful if the doctor will sometimes give feedback to the patient about what the doctor has heard and understands. Some patients get a better understanding of themselves and what they want to do just by talking to an empathic, nonjudgmental person. Clarification and reality testing are frequently used. By helping the patient to clarify thoughts and feelings and by occasionally pointing out reality, the doctor can aid in this understanding. With supportive therapy one tries to help the patient recapture self-esteem and to utilize their coping mechanisms to best advantage. For example, one encourages a patient who is highly intellectual to use this ability to better understand how to proceed with problem solving.

One who is not trained in psychotherapy should not, however, attempt the kind of psychotherapy that deals with unconscious conflicts and past relationships. The danger in attempting this is that it will stir up feelings that neither the patient nor the therapist can handle. The patient may become more upset instead of resolving problems.

Doctors can usually avoid becoming too deeply entangled by following a few guidelines. Interviews that are primarily for supportive psychotherapy should be kept to a prescribed length of time and not allowed to run indefinitely. Twenty or thirty minutes would be a reasonable time for these follow-up interviews. Frequency of the interviews is important in titrating the intensity of the relationship. Patients who come in quite frequently over a period of time may develop such an intense relationship as to impair or negate the help the doctor is trying to provide. Therefore, interviews should not be more than once a week and should not extend regularly over a long period. If it appears that it will take a long time to resolve a problem, psychiatric consultation should be sought. Many patients will receive much help by being seen intermittently. Intermittent visits may be extended over a longer period of time.

It is best to keep the discussion focused on the patient's present situation and oriented to attitudes, feelings, and problems about current reality. The past can be discussed, but the interviews should not dwell on the past, and the patient should be helped to return to the present.

Advice can, and should, be given about medical matters. Sometimes advice about relaxation techniques and stress management is helpful. It is best to avoid, as much as possible, giving advice about psychosocial issues such as how to handle family problems. Instead, help the patient to view possible alternatives. With these guidelines in mind, a doctor should be helpful to the patient without becoming too deeply entwined in a relationship that may ultimately prove harmful to the patient.

Does psychotherapy work? For a moving account of psychotherapy and an answer to the question, the reader is referred to Hannah Green's *I Never Promised You a Rose Garden* (1964). Growth toward maturity is an inherent trait in every individual. Some have called it a drive for self-actualization (Goldstein 1939). Many biological, psychological, and social impediments to self-actualization arise during one's lifetime. Psychotherapy aids the patient in removing the psychological impediments. The psychiatric evaluation is the first step in assessing all the impediments. An important part of the evaluation is to gather information about content and feelings as they relate to a patient's present problems and past life. This can be therapeutic for the patient, even in the initial interviews.

In the following account, the highlights of approximately three years of psychotherapy are presented, during which a patient with an accepting therapist could relive childhood feelings, come to understand and take responsibility for these feelings, and finally try new ways of relating to the outside world. Much of the material is presented in the patient's own words because she portrays her feelings and the process of therapy so eloquently.

The present illness for this 36-year-old woman began about four years before beginning long-term psychotherapy. She was divorced, moved to another city, and was doing well on her job until she had an automobile accident. There was no apparent injury from the accident.

She was seen and immediately discharged from an emergency room; however, she began to have difficulty with her memory, dizziness, blackouts, and trouble with her speech. Her job performance deteriorated to the point that she was finally discharged by her employer. She became so depressed and anxious that she was admitted to the psychiatric unit of a general hospital. There she was placed on psychotropic medication. She improved and was discharged to a psychiatry outpatient clinic where she was seen intermittently for support and to monitor her medication. Because her memory and speech problems persisted, organic brain syndrome was suspected. For this reason she was admitted for a neurological evaluation, which showed no organic brain disease. During an interview using sodium amytal in the hospital, she was able to speak clearly. After being discharged she remained anxious and depressed, so the minor tranquilizer and an antidepressant prescribed in the hospital were continued.

An attractive, but heavily made up, anxious woman came to the first psychotherapy interview. She stuttered and had trouble finding the right word. At times, during the interview she would get so nervous that her hands and feet would shake. She could remember little of her past life.

During the first months she complained about how hard it was to come to therapy. She had trouble remembering the way, but she usually arrived early for each session. While in the waiting room she would pace and chain smoke. She said that she could not trust the therapist and, therefore, could not say what was on her mind. She avoided talking about feelings, would stutter, and say she couldn't remember.

During one interview she became extremely angry with the therapist, who had been late to several sessions. The patient said that the therapist didn't appreciate her. Following this outburst the patient became fearful that the therapist would not want to see her anymore, but she was reassured that the therapist would be there for her next appointment. For several more sessions she was both angry and suspicious. She would scream at the therapist for not helping her and talk about how much her family had mistreated her.

Usually she came in neatly and modestly dressed, but one day she came in with fancy boots and decorated tight pants. She began talking about her two personalities. One was a trim, proper, self-effacing lady. The other was an aggressive woman of the world. She was told by others that at times she would dress in her tight pants and be hostile to everyone, but afterwards she wouldn't remember having done so.

The patient said,

> This other person didn't come out until I had the accident. It's like I would black out. I wasn't there for a while. I'm not trying

to blame it on another person. It's a real strong personality that comes out of me. I thought it had left and gone away, but evidently she . . . she. I know it's me. It's just another personality. I'm not trying to blame it on another person

The therapist asked her how she felt about it and she said, "It really scares me. That other woman scares me." But, in spite of her fear, she was beginning to accept her own hostility and aggression, and as this occurred she allowed herself to become more deeply involved in therapy.

I began to realize that when I am here with you (the therapist) that this is my hour. I just thought about it the other day and it occurred to me that I am wasting my time by taking things so lightly here. I should get more deeply into my emotional problems and say what's bothering me.

You know, at one time in therapy, in the beginning, I didn't like you at all. For many months I tried not to respond and not get anxious, but deep down inside I wanted to yell "help me." At this time I thought I was going crazy and would end up behind bars in a mental hospital.

I found myself coming to see you although I didn't really trust you. On the other hand, in another part of my personality, I thought you would protect me. I wanted you to protect me from the goblins and things, those figments of my imagination.

But then I found myself coming and saying "This is how I feel" and telling you what is really bothering me. Now I feel like I'm at the bottom of a ten-story building and I'm trying to climb the staircase. I take two steps forward and one step back, but that one step is the most important.

The patient wanted to go to college or vocational school. She couldn't decide which one, but she made tentative steps in both directions and felt rebuffed. She took on a part-time job and did well, but had the feeling that some of the people she worked with didn't like her work. Nevertheless, in spite of her misgivings she was willing to try new behavior. Later in therapy she said, "Now I realize it wasn't them, it was me. I have to be responsible for my own actions."

As months went on she began getting along better with her family, but she still came in with heavy makeup and a meticulous hairdo. She continued to take large doses of the minor tranquilizer. Finally, she began to accept the therapist's suggestion that she begin reducing the dose of her medication. One day she came in with short hair. She began to smile more and talked spontaneously. Toward the end of therapy she talked about her personality change.

It's like seeing the world for the first time. Every day I wake up to something new. It's a wonderful experience. I never thought I'd be in this position. I started out taking something in the hospital that I thought was harmless years ago. Something to calm me down. It made me drunk, but it felt so good. Then I started taking the tranquilizer. It gave me the courage to be this sophisticated, worldly woman I thought I wanted to be.

When I began to stop taking the tranquilizer it really had to do with acceptance of my mother's death when I was a little girl. I think it went back to my childhood. She died when she was 35 years old, and when I was 35 years old, I wanted to stop taking the tranquilizer because I accepted that she was dead—that she had died. She was 35 years old when she died and that was the age I had to be to start living.

I took on two personalities fifteen years ago. It all went back to when my mother died and it had to do with my stepmother. I was four years old when my mother died. I was very alone. It's pretty complicated. After she died, my father married another woman and I was glad to get her. I had asked God to bring my mother back. He didn't, but he brought me a stepmother. Then she left. So, when I was a young lady, I took the role that I thought she was—my fantasies of her. I dyed my hair and began to smoke and tried to look sophisticated.

Then I think I saw you in the role of my mother. When I was a girl, I used to imagine that women I liked were Mother. Even after I grew up, I would see a woman and imagine her as a mother.

Since in my mind I had you in the same role as my mother, then I had to trust you in the same way as my mother—when I was a little girl—to give up the tranquilizer. That night I called you up I wanted you to help me see something. I kept thinking "She knows what it is. Why doesn't she tell me?" You said, "When you're ready to see it, you will." That night I saw a coffin with purple velvet and I cried because my mother was dead— she was finally dead and I wasn't bitter anymore.

Now I get up and see a beautiful world. I jog a mile a day. I'm going back to school and I don't need anybody to do my thinking for me.

References

Alexander F, French TM: *Psychoanalytic Therapy: Principles and Application.* New York, Ronald Press, 1946.

Frank JD: An overview of psychotherapy, in Usdin G (ed): *Overview of the Psychotherapies.* New York, Brunner/Mazel, 1975.

Goldstein K: *The Organism*. New York, American Book, 1939.

Green H: *I Never Promised You a Rose Garden*. New York, Holt Rinehart & Winston, 1964.

Karasu TB (chairperson): *The Psychiatric Therapies*. The American Psychiatric Association Commission on Psychiatric Therapies. Washington, DC, American Psychiatric Association, 1984.

Suggested Reading

Bruch H: *Learning Psychotherapy*. Cambridge, Harvard University Press, 1974.

14

An Organizing Framework

In closing, I would like to provide the reader with a broad frame of reference with which to think about and organize information from and about psychiatric patients, and into which one can fit more specific theories and show how they relate. With such a vast amount of data pouring in from laboratory and other tests, physical examination, interviews with patient and family, and information about the culture and environment, we need a way to organize it.

Implicitly or explicitly everyone has a notion, hypothesis, or theory about what causes another person to act as he or she does. One of the problems medical students and physicians have with psychiatry in contrast to, for example, biochemistry or internal medicine is that the organizing theories they use to understand mental patients are often nonscientific folk dogmas or prejudices, or material from their unconscious. It is much more difficult to bring such dogmas and prejudices to the study of biochemistry because the data and knowledge base of biochemistry does not fall within the everyday experience of the family and the culture. Thus, one does not grow up being indoctrinated with ideas and information that seem to relate to that science. However, each of us has lived and so, mistakenly, believes he or she is an expert in the realm of human emotions and behavior. The student must use the feelings and thoughts he or she experiences to help understand patients. But these are not to be used indiscriminately, even if the doctor truly believes that what is being done is in the patient's best interest. If the doctor has an organizing theory into which to fit data and hypotheses and on which to base actions, then feelings will not serve as an indiscriminate stimulus for action.

The value of a frame of reference is in the way it helps the mind to analyze perceptions and data. Everyone has a frame of reference, whether or not he or she is aware of it. In science, they change and evolve as new knowledge and theory come to the fore. This is not so with prejudice and dogma where facts have little impact on beliefs. The science of human behavior has evolved from myth and dogma as have other sciences, but it has evolved more recently, it is more complex than other sciences, and it lacks the precision instruments for studying the various phenomena. Therefore, we find that dogma and myth tend to creep back into our thinking about human behavior more often than in our thinking about other natural sciences.

In the past, human behavior, good and bad, was ascribed to some supernatural power. The mentally ill were often thought to be possessed by some evil. This type of thinking reached notorious extremes during the Inquisition of the sixteenth and seventeenth centuries. At that time, the symptoms of the mentally ill were attributed to witchcraft. Those possessed were tortured and burned to rid them of the devil's influence. The Inquisition was, of course, also an instrument of political power, and all who were disposed of by the Star Chamber were not mentally ill. But the mentally ill were and still are an easy mark for unscrupulous politicians. The ravages of the Inquisition also spilled over into the New World. Early European settlers in America would subject their fellow citizens to horrible tortures to drive out this devil that was supposed to be causing unacceptable behavior or evil thoughts. Not everyone, of course, even in those times, accepted the devil as an explanation for deviant behavior, but those who did would listen to a troubled person with that particular belief and would evaluate all that was heard in terms of such an erroneous theory.

Today's society is by no means immune to those who would use dogmatism and demagoguery to gain control over the minds and behavior of others. A cult leader brings hundreds into the jungles of South America where they die of self-inflicted poison. Various self-proclaimed moral leaders try to inject themselves into the political system of a country in order to control what they have decreed to be decadent thinking and behavior. Fortunately, today rational thinking tends to predominate, although sometimes only by a slim margin.

The absence of free will was another concept often invoked to explain deviant behavior. People who did not do what those in authority thought was right were said to be lacking will power. Showing them the consequences of their behavior would presumably restore their will. Interestingly, some of the same methods used to drive out the devil—dunking, spinning, locking up—were also used to help restore will power. Only this time there was a different theory of causation. We could, of course, speculate that the basic motive in all of this was to exert power and influence in a hostile manner upon other humans, but the examination of such motives is beyond the scope of this book.

The nineteenth century saw a series of major efforts on many fronts to investigate scientifically the inner workings of the mind and the determinants of human behavior. Three major areas of investigation— biological, psychological, and social—began at that time and each still contributes to our understanding of mental illness. Each has its own body of knowledge and methods of investigation. We gather data from patients in each of these areas. To help our patients best we need some way to organize this data.

One broad organizing theory is general systems theory, out of which arises the biopsychosocial model of medical practice. A brief general description should give the reader an overall organizing frame of reference to aid in the collection and organization of data. A preliminary word of caution: General systems theory and the biopsychosocial model are broad organizing concepts. They are so broad as to be compared, say, with one's outlook on life, or, perhaps, with whether one is Republican or Democrat, or whether one has been brought up in the Judeo–Christian or the Buddhist tradition. General systems theory, however, deals with scientifically derived information. As with all such broad concepts, they must be related to more narrowly defined subsystems that explain specific phenomena.

To explain human behavior, we must have knowledge of physical, psychological, and social functions. General systems theory helps us understand their relationship to explain a patient's behavior. Von Bertalanffy (1968), one of the original developers of general systems theory, describes it as follows:

> General system theory, therefore, is a general science of "wholeness" which up till now was considered a vague, hazy, and semimetaphysical concept. In elaborate form it would be a logicomathematical discipline, in itself purely formal but applicable to various empirical sciences. For sciences concerned with "organized wholes," it would be of similar significance to that which probability theory has for sciences concerned with "chance events;" the latter, too, is a formal mathematical discipline which can be applied to most diverse fields, such as thermodynamics, biological and medical experimentation, genetics, life insurance statistics, etc.

The universe is composed of a large, but apparently finite number of systems from the subatomic to the cosmic. Each system has important interactions with adjacent and related systems and each exerts some influence, albeit small in some cases, on all other systems. Furthermore, there are numerous hierarchies of systems. Atoms are themselves a system. They form the building blocks of molecules, a separate and more complex system. The type of atoms in a molecule help to determine, but do not solely determine, the properties of a compound, because a compound is a system of its own with a more complex structure. Compounds will react with one another and the type of reaction will be determined by the properties and the structure of the compounds, which are in turn partly determined by the component atoms. The product developed from the reaction of compounds could become the component of a cell or an airplane, which are other orders of systems. *Systems theory recognizes simple and complex systems, their hierarchies, and presents a way to observe and study them scientifically. Systems theory helps to prevent thinking only in terms of isolated, segregated entities.*

The biopsychosocial model is a systems approach to understanding a person and the relationship of systems outside and inside of that person that influence health and illness. A brief explanation of the biopsychosocial model in the context of general systems theory provides a broad frame to guide explorations and to understand information obtained. For a more detailed explanation the reader is referred to Engel's "The Clinical Application of the Biopsychosocial Model" (1980). The biopsychosocial model of illness attempts to develop a conceptual model including all the factors that impinge upon a patient and contribute to his or her illness. In this way, it differs from a biomedical model which views a smaller number of systems and may ignore others. The biomedical model looks at the disease in a person: "the hepatitis in Room 4." The biopsychosocial model views the whole person, including the disease processes and how the illness may relate to the patient's personality and the society in which he or she lives.

The biopsychosocial model would take into account that the patient with hepatitis might be a heroin addict. With this frame of reference the physician would inquire into the patient's psychosocial history to learn about early family life and socioeconomic circumstances that may have contributed to the patient's becoming an addict. With this information, the doctor can better understand and help the patient through the treatment of the acute illness and help develop, with the patient, a long-range treatment plan. This might lead the patient to a change of lifestyle and even prevent an untimely death from an overdose or from AIDS.

We know more about some systems than about others. We usually have more information about relationships within a system than relationships among systems. We can quantify hemoglobin and red blood cells in the determination of anemia. We can quantify the income level that defines poverty that contributes to an iron-deficiency anemia. It is more difficult to quantify those aspects of culture and society that influence eating habits or infant feeding as to produce an iron-deficiency anemia. True, we can measure the iron in the food intake, but how do you measure a belief system that refuses to change even in the face of demonstrated fact? Yet all are equally important if we are to understand the patient's illness and prescribe proper treatment.

Using the biopsychosocial model as a frame of reference, such diverse factors can be put into perspective. The physician can evaluate organic pathophysiological processes, mental processes, and the social situation and culture that may be influencing the patient. The significant interaction of all important findings from all systems are then evaluated for their relative importance in the patient's presenting problem.

The basic reference for the physician is the patient. What is learned from the social system and how the patient reacts to it is referred back to his or her feelings and behavior. What is learned of a cell's pathophysiology is important for its ultimate impact on the feelings, thoughts, and behavior and total functioning of the person. With the person as the central focus, one can range widely in gathering information, keeping in mind various theoretical orientations for applying the knowledge gained to the feeling, thinking, behaving person.

Engel (1980) gives an example of a patient admitted to the hospital with acute myocardial infarction who was doing well, but suddenly developed cardiac arrest attributable to an inept attempt to obtain a sample of arterial blood. It was not the drawing of blood per se that caused the arrest but the feelings that the patient had about the procedure. These feelings, in turn, set in motion a chain of physiologic events that culminated in ventricular fibrillation. At another time or with another patient, the procedure might not have started this chain of events. The important thing was the meaning to the patient at that time.

If physicians choose to ignore the psychological meaning of what is going on around the patient and its interaction with physiologic systems, they may well be jeopardizing their patient's health. The physician will not be treating the whole patient nor will he or she be a whole physician.

General systems theory and the biopsychosocial model are broad concepts by which one may order a wide variety of data; they are not sufficiently precise in themselves to explain specific phenomena. The theory and the model offer a way of relating systems. Other constructs are necessary to explain phenomena within a system or subsystem. For example, a body of data and theory explains what happens within the cardiovascular system, including data from other systems such as the cellular and endocrine system. The biopsychosocial model helps to relate data from these systems to data from the psychological and social system.

Just as we need data and theory to explain what happens within the cardiovascular system, we need theory to explain what we observe from the psychological system. Numerous theories explain thinking, feeling, and behavior. The most useful at present are developmental theories and learning theory. Most useful theories of emotional development are derived from psychoanalytic theory. These include concepts of the unconscious, basic instincts, and ego development. Using observations based on sociology and anthropology, some psychoanalysts, notably Erikson (1963), have developed useful constructs that relate ego development to culture and society.

"Psychoanalysis, for example, uncovers a realm of the unconscious which is not observed in naive experience. In order to explain what is observed, both physics and psychology construct models and theoretical systems which greatly surpass immediate experience and are linked with the latter only by long chains of deductive reasoning" (von Bertalanffy 1964).

Piaget (1969) was the master observer and theoretician in the area of cognitive development. Children's cognitive abilities to perceive, analyze, and understand the world about them profoundly influence their emotional development. To understand any particular developmental stage, one cannot neglect its cognitive development.

Learning theory, is useful in understanding specific behavior. The concepts of reinforcement or reward, extinction, and punishment frequently help to explain observed patient actions. Learning theory does not in itself explain emotional and cognitive developmental process.

Ideally, we should have one theory to explain feeling, thinking, and observed behavior. The science of human behavior is not yet so well advanced, but using developmental and learning theory concepts along with knowledge of biology, culture, and society, one can begin to explain psychological and behavioral phenomena in psychiatric patients. These phenomena have their origins in an organic brain and, through the brain, influence other organ systems within the body for better or worse. Here in the specifics of these systems' interaction lie the nuts and bolts of the biopsychosocial model. The essential principle is to keep various components and systems in mind. We currently have no way to quantitate the interaction of these systems, so observation and experience must be our guide.

As the observer gets farther from the system under direct study and looks at related systems, the degree of certainty becomes less and the degree of approximation becomes greater. By studying a patient's symptoms we can be fairly certain of the diagnosis. In psychiatry, we investigate present illness and past history, family relationships, genetic and predisposing factors, and related organic conditions and try to make an approximation of the etiology and pathogenesis of the disorder. The degree of certainty with which we integrate all of these factors is less than the degree of certainty with which we make the diagnosis. Prognosis that involves some prediction is another matter and an even greater approximation.

> In practical terms the doctor's tasks are, first, to find out *how* and *what* the patient is or has been feeling and experiencing; then to formulate explanations (hypotheses) for the patient's feelings and experiences (the "why" and the "what for"); to engage the patient's participation in further clinical and laboratory studies to test such hypotheses; and, finally, to elicit the patient's co-operation in activities aimed to alleviate distress and/or correct underlying derangements that may be contributing to distress or disability. The patient's tasks and responsibilities complement those of the physician (Engel 1980).

In the biopsychosocial model, the doctor–patient relationship is one of the main tools for evaluation and therapy. Knowledge must be acquired and skills must be polished in this area just as one learns physical diagnosis and, later, complicated surgical techniques. The cardiologist must learn to palpate and percuss the chest, listen to the heart, read a cardiogram and, as he or she progresses, to learn even more complicated diagnostic procedures. So it is with the interpersonal skills of medicine. Finally, putting it all together for the benefit of the patient is the art and science of medicine.

Daniel Carleton Gajdusek received the Nobel Prize in Medicine for what is probably one of the best examples of the use of the biopsychosocial model in medical research. In his study of kuru, a progressive degeneration of the nervous system, he not only determined that the disease was due to a slow virus that took years to produce its clinical effects, but he also was able to determine that the virus was transmitted as a result of a highly specific, culturally determined ritual involving cannibalism of relatives who had just died. During the ritualistic eating, children were contaminated with the kuru virus, and they would later develop symptoms. Knowing the etiology and pathophysiology of kuru would have done little for the victims of the disease if the cultural mode of transmission were not also known. Gajdusek is an unusual person: a virologist, anthropologist, linguist, and world traveler, among other things. As a person, he embodies the biopsychosocial model (Gajdusek 1977).

The biopsychosocial model is a systems approach to the person. It includes the various systems within and without that person that influence his or her health. This book concentrates most on the psychological and social systems because we are approaching interviewing with that in mind, but that does not mean that physiochemical systems are not equally important. Medicine has advanced spectacularly in this area in the last century, and spectacular advances in this area will continue. The scientist in the laboratory must, necessarily, be preoccupied with the physiochemical mechanisms of disease.

With the biopsychosocial model as an organizing concept, the interviewer is free to follow patients as they begin to explore what is troubling them. The doctor can comfortably range widely with the patient if this proves necessary, secure in the knowledge that he or she has some organizing principles to relate the data. In one of the interviews that we used for illustration, the reader followed a patient through such disparate events as drugs and drinking, a divorce, a war-time city, and a Gulf Coast hurricane.

In many of the other interviews illustrating certain points or techniques, physical problems relate to mental states, both of which may be inextricably entwined with environmental situations. If we consider all of these in light of the theoretic structure discussed, we can gather information about physical illness and the various bodily systems. We can hear about a strained relationship with a daughter-in-law and about fears of being abandoned—with the knowledge that, although we are gathering what seems to be unrelated information, it will fall within one system or another and that the systems themselves have a meaningful and often potent interaction.

An international event triggering an upheaval in the social system which then upsets a significant other (spouse, for example) can produce feelings (brain) that will stimulate a physiologic response, which will affect a target organ, such as the digestive system, to exacerbate a duodenal ulcer. To be more specific, a Mexican American woman married to an illegal alien develops asthma when her husband is deported to Mexico. An international incident precipitates an illness.

References

Engel G: The clinical application of the biopsychosocial model. *Am J Psychiatry* 1980;137:535–543.

Erikson EK: *Childhood and Society*, 2d ed. New York, Norton, 1963.

Gajdusek DC: Unconventional viruses and the origin and disappearance of kuru. *Science* 1977;197:943–960.

Piaget J, Inhelder B: *The Psychology of the Child*. New York, Basic Books, 1969.

Von Bertalanffy L: The mind–body problem: a new view. *Psychosom Med* 1964;26:29–45.

Von Bertalanffy L: *General Systems Theory*. New York, Braziller, 1968.

15

Epilogue:
A Short Interview

This interview was conducted by the author with a woman who was bringing her children to a small neighborhood pediatric clinic. A group of six first-year medical students were assigned to the clinic to study the families of children brought there. The woman agreed to be interviewed in front of the group. The purpose of the interview was to help the students learn more about personal and family problems of families who bring children to the clinic and to illustrate interviewing technique.

This interview was selected for several reasons. It illustrates how patients are willing to talk about their problems when given the opportunity. Furthermore, this was not an interview in the doctor's private office but was carried out before a group of several students in a not-so-private room of a busy clinic. The woman begins by discussing some problems her daughter is having. With some encouragement, she begins discussing her own problems and then discusses the interpersonal and intrapsychic dynamics that contribute to these problems.

Many of the elements discussed in this book are illustrated in this short interview: techniques used in helping the patient talk about things most important to her, the importance of feelings in illness and current problems, and the importance of past history. The interview is taken verbatim from a videotape except for some parts, left out in the interest of brevity. The pauses and some of the feeling tone do not come through when written. Otherwise the words are as spoken.

DOCTOR: Did the nurse tell you what this was about?

PATIENT: Yes, it was an interview about, something about the background of the family . . .

DOCTOR: That's right.

PATIENT: Sicknesses, whatever we had.

DOCTOR: Sickness and what your problems are. We just like to know in general about your family. So, maybe you could start out by telling us how many children you have, who come to the clinic here.

PATIENT: I have six and there's only one that I'm bringing over here to this clinic.

DOCTOR: Six children. What ages are your children?

PATIENT: From 17 to this one that I have, 3 years and 1 month.

DOCTOR: And this is the youngest that you're bringing to the clinic?

PATIENT: Yes.

DOCTOR: And is your 17-year-old in high school, through high school?

PATIENT: No, she dropped out early. (Laughs)

DOCTOR: When did she drop out?

PATIENT: This year.

DOCTOR: What grade was she in?

PATIENT: Tenth.

DOCTOR: Tenth grade. What is she doing?

PATIENT: Oh, just around the house.

DOCTOR: Um hm. Is she working?

PATIENT: No, she don't work. She just stays around the house and helps with the house chores.

(Until now this interview seems to have violated most of the rules propounded in this book and, in essence, it has. There are many direct questions requiring short answers. Nevertheless, during this time a relationship is being established, a feeling tone is developing and the patient is becoming more comfortable. The questions and answers are a means to an end, not an end in themselves. You recall that we said that the doctor must, early in the interview [and by early I mean immediately], appraise the emotional tone of the interview and react accordingly.

The ability to appreciate the emotional tone of an interview can be learned and become explicit in the interviewer's mind; however, those who do it best have a native ability. Halfbacks who can run through the opposing football team, sensing their opponents' moves before they occur, conduct some of the best interviews I have seen.)

DOCTOR: How do you feel about that?

("How do you feel about that?" changes the tone and the type of interaction.)

PATIENT: Well, at first I couldn't stand for her to be at home because I wanted her to be back in school. I didn't want her to be a dropout. I wanted her to finish school. But, then she just said that she didn't want to go anymore. And I know it might be because she's overweight. I think that's her problem. I don't know for sure. She'll be 17 the 20th of this month.

DOCTOR: Yeah.

PATIENT: And she weighs over 300 pounds.

DOCTOR: Three hundred pounds. So she is quite a bit overweight.

PATIENT: Um hm. She's just a little bit taller than I am.

DOCTOR: How long has she had this problem of being so overweight?

PATIENT: She started being like that since she was around 15.

DOCTOR: About 15. And before that, was she a little bit overweight or not at all?

PATIENT: No, well, I could say that she was just normal weight. We never know until they get to the age of 15 what kind of shape they're going to have and all that. Like she's the only one that's overweight.

DOCTOR: She's the only one with that problem. When she was 15 she started getting overweight?

PATIENT: I don't know if that's when it started, but I think it was because that's when I noticed she was getting fatter.

DOCTOR: Um hm. Do you see that as a pretty big problem, yourself, I mean?

PATIENT: Well, I do think it is a problem.

DOCTOR: That makes it hard for her in school?

PATIENT: Um hm. Because I've been trying to make her go out to work. Well, she says that she's afraid to travel in buses and all that, and that's the only transportation she can get.

DOCTOR: What is she afraid of?

PATIENT: That's another thing that I don't know.

DOCTOR: You don't know. She's afraid. And you think that she was feeling badly about going to school because of her overweightness?

PATIENT: Um hm.

DOCTOR: Do you have any idea about why somebody would get overweight like that? I notice that you're a little bit overweight yourself, right?

(The earlier comments by the doctor were in part to encourage the woman to mention her own obesity. It was obviously a major problem, which had to be addressed at some point in the interview. Not to acknowledge the obvious fact of obesity would have impaired the relationship. Notice what happens when the obesity is made explicit.)

PATIENT: And I've come down already.

DOCTOR: Oh, really?

PATIENT: I used to weigh 310 pounds.

DOCTOR: Oh my!

PATIENT: But then I went to the doctor because I started to feel sick and all that.

DOCTOR: Yeah . . .

PATIENT: High blood pressure and all that.

DOCTOR: Yeah . . .

PATIENT: And so they started giving me medicines and I started on my own to stop eating and all that and I noticed that I've lost weight.

DOCTOR: Well, you've done pretty . . . how much do you weigh now? Do you know?

PATIENT: I weigh 273.

DOCTOR: So you've lost quite a bit already. And do you plan to lose some more?

PATIENT: I hope so.

DOCTOR: Very good. Well, you know a little bit about this overweight problem then, don't you?

PATIENT: Yeah.

DOCTOR: Tell me about it. I mean, what would cause somebody like you or your daughter to get . . .

PATIENT: Well on me, talking for myself, I'd say that what has been getting me overweight was that since my baby was born, that since he was born, you know, I had to have an operation for him to be born, so. . . .

DOCTOR: I see, that was the last one?

PATIENT: Yeah. Because the youngest child was 9 by the time I got this one. So, that's when I started just laying around and being lazy—just letting everybody work and for myself just laying around. So, all I worried about was to eat and sleep and sit down and look at T.V. and all that.

DOCTOR: Well, you must have had some worries to do that, or things that were making you feel blue—something like that?

(This comment, "You must have had some worries . . ." illustrates the importance of having some theory to guide one's operations. Using the theory that all behavior is determined by underlying emotions and conflicts, the interviewer did not accept the statement that this woman was lazy. "Lazy" is simply a lay descriptive term for inactivity. We presume that there are underlying personality dynamics responsible for this behavior.)

PATIENT: Well, the main trouble was that my daughter, that's when she stopped going to school. Once she used to go and then she didn't want to go, and she started going back, and then she didn't want to go anymore, and then . . . well, my mother would take over because she's the kind of grandmother that will stick up for her grandchildren and she don't want the mother to hit them or anything. And so, I just think that my problem is in my own home. Because I started worrying and I started quarreling with her and all that. And by the time I knew it, that's when I started feeling that I was hungry because I made too much appetite working out, talking, walking back and forth.

(As with many patients, she has some idea of why she overeats. She knows it has something to do with feeling depressed and angry.)

DOCTOR: I see.

PATIENT: And then, after that I just let everything go, just forgot about everything.

DOCTOR: In other words, you were, now if I understood you right, you and your mother were having trouble and she was kind of taking over with the kids. Is that right?

PATIENT: Um hm.

DOCTOR: And you were getting angry with her?

PATIENT: I guess that was my main problem.

DOCTOR: Um hm. These are the medical students we told you about.

(This interview was chosen in part to illustrate how a relationship can develop with patient and doctor in spite of distraction. The patient was told that more students might come in during the interview. The interviewer then summed up the previous discussion for the students.)

DOCTOR: (To students) We were talking to Mrs. G about her oldest daughter right now—her oldest daughter is 17 and has dropped out of school and has got a problem. She's overweight. She weighs what? Over 200 pounds?

PATIENT: She weighs over 300 pounds.

DOCTOR: Mrs. G was saying too that she was having a problem with overweightness, so we were talking about what causes somebody to be overweight . . . eat too much, huh?

PATIENT: (Laughs) I guess so.

DOCTOR: And you were saying that your, let's see, that was right after your last child was born, and he's now how old?

PATIENT: Three.

DOCTOR: And you had to have that operation for the baby to be born? And then you and your mother were having some difficulty, more so than you used to have?

PATIENT: Um hm.

DOCTOR: I see. And has she been living with you all the time?

PATIENT: Well, she's been living with me for about five years now, you know, steady. We've been living in the same house, so, I don't know, maybe what my worry was was that I was afraid for her to take over everything, including the kids.

DOCTOR: Yeah, and she would like to do that?

PATIENT: I guess so.

DOCTOR: Or she tries to do that?

PATIENT: Well sometimes she does, but then she don't.

DOCTOR: I see. You're afraid she might do that?

PATIENT: Well, sometimes I am.

DOCTOR: What sort of feelings do you have inside about that?

(This demonstrates how a general question about feelings may open another dimension for discussion.)

PATIENT: Well, once I started to worry because I used to think that she was going to take over and I would be left alone all by myself. She doesn't have nobody anymore, just me, and my brothers are all in Chicago, and all of them are, you know, separated from their wives and everything; so, uh, I guess what she needed was just company; and it's like I say, well, like now, I don't have any hard feelings against her or nothing. I just let everything go, and if she talks, I just let her talk.

DOCTOR: You don't get angry?

PATIENT: No, not any more.

DOCTOR: What makes the difference from what it used to be?

PATIENT: I don't know. Maybe it's because I got used to it or . . . I think that's the main thing; I got used to it.

DOCTOR: But you were afraid that she was going to take over?

PATIENT: Before?

DOCTOR: And kind of take all your kids away from you?

PATIENT: Um hm.

DOCTOR: And then you'd be all by yourself with not anybody to take care of or be with you?

PATIENT: No . . . I was afraid to be by myself—that I was going to stay by myself.

DOCTOR: You mean you were afraid she was really going to take the kids out of the home?

PATIENT: Um hm.

DOCTOR: Oh, I see. So that's what was upsetting you a lot.

PATIENT: Um hm.

DOCTOR: And it started when she moved in with you.

PATIENT: Um hm. 'Cause, like I could say that she took over my two oldest kids because they won't do what I say; they'll do what she says.

DOCTOR: Um hm.

PATIENT: And . . . they were from my first marriage, and then the other three, they don't follow her, they just follow me, everywhere I go, they go with me.

DOCTOR: Um hm.

PATIENT: So, that's what made me feel good. I still have somebody to follow me.

DOCTOR: But you had to find that out.

PATIENT: Yeah. (Laughs)

DOCTOR: That must have been a pretty hard time for you.

PATIENT: At first it was, but then, like I say . . .

DOCTOR: Once you learned that she wasn't going to take them all, it was a little better.

PATIENT: Um hm.

DOCTOR: How much did you weigh before she moved in?

PATIENT: Uh, I was 190.

DOCTOR: One ninety. And then you got up to 300 pounds. And

how long did it take you to get that far? 'Til you got up over 300 pounds yourself, you said, didn't you?

PATIENT: Um hm. I guess it was about nine months or a year.

DOCTOR: Um hm. And that time was when you were worried and upset and you said you were pacing the floor and you'd go and eat.

PATIENT: Yeah. Because at that time she was mad at me because I married for the third time because she didn't like my husband because he was an illegal alien, you know, and so she didn't like the idea of me getting married to the father of my baby, and she said she didn't want me at home anymore.

(Here the interviewer finds out factual information without specifically asking, just by encouraging the patient to talk.)

DOCTOR: I see, oh . . .

PATIENT: So, all those things, you know . . . everything came together at the same time.

DOCTOR: Oh my gosh, yeah. And you had the baby and you had to have a caesarean section for that, and then you got married at the same time, and your mother talked like she was going to throw you out.

PATIENT: Um hm.

DOCTOR: It's pretty frightening, isn't it?

PATIENT: It sure is!

DOCTOR: But it was your house.

PATIENT: It was my house, and still, well, like right now, if I do something she don't like, well, I get kicked out of it (laughs). But then, it's like I say, like I don't worry any more, 'cause like now, right now, I have help from welfare and my late husband's pension and, you know, social security, and well, it's like if she kicks me out, well she can keep the house anyway; I have money to rent another one.

DOCTOR: But she can kick you out if she wants to, even if it's your house?

PATIENT: (Laughs) Yeah, and I don't say anything about it because it's all right.

DOCTOR: You don't say anything about it.

(This is all incomprehensible without some organizing theory. Why is she so passive as to allow her mother to throw her out? Why doesn't she express some feelings about the prospect—specifically anger? The reader is referred to books on obesity and on personality theory. Obesity and dependency often go together. Dependent people tend to be passive and repress their hostility.)

PATIENT: Yes, because she's pretty old.

DOCTOR: She's pretty old? How old is she?

PATIENT: Oh, 58 . . . 57 or 58.

DOCTOR: Oh.

PATIENT: But she has diabetes, you know. She's been nervous and everything.

DOCTOR: So you're really kind of afraid to upset her any more. Is that what you're telling us?

PATIENT: Um hm.

DOCTOR: So you've got your mother you're afraid to upset and all these kids to take care of, huh?

PATIENT: Yeah (laughs).

DOCTOR: What do you do for yourself?

PATIENT: Uh . . . like?

DOCTOR: Well, like to get something out of your life, that you enjoy.

PATIENT: Well, like when I feel worried and all that, I take the kids out to the park and we go around down here and have some fun, and we stay out there all day, and in the evening we come back home and we get to eat and look at T.V. and go to sleep.

DOCTOR: Do you have a car?

PATIENT: Um hm.

DOCTOR: Well that's good. That helps.

PATIENT: Um hm.

DOCTOR: How about you? Do you get out yourself?

PATIENT: Well once in a while. I like to go dancing.

DOCTOR: Are you married now?

PATIENT: No. I divorced my husband because, after he came back from Mexico and I got him a passport and everything, he just took off and I never saw him again.

DOCTOR: Oh, he was in the country illegally at first when you first married him. Is that right?

PATIENT: Um hm.

DOCTOR: And then you helped him go back?

PATIENT: Well, we stayed here after the baby was born. I met him before, after I was having trouble with my mother. Well he said he was going to help me out and give me a home of my own and everything. So, I just said, all right, I'll take a chance and see because maybe I'll be a little bit happier then. And so I said, well, okay. When the baby was born, that's when we took off and went to Mexico and got married over there and came back and he started, you know, trying to get his passport and everything. After that he got it and I went back there and brought him back and so, when he got here he went somewhere up North. And he said he was going to write from there and send for me and he didn't. And so, by the time I knew it, I waited for six months and in six months he didn't come back. Then I got a Legal Aid attorney and told him what happened and everything and that I wanted a divorce and they gave it to me.

DOCTOR: So that's another disappointment in your life, huh?

PATIENT: Um hm.

DOCTOR: You've had a lot of those, haven't you?

PATIENT: Quite a bit.

DOCTOR: What other ones have you had?

PATIENT: Well, starting from when I started to have my second child; well, my husband was . . . the train killed him. That was way before, when my second child was born.

DOCTOR: A train killed him? Was he working for the railroad?

PATIENT: Um . . . no, he was working for _____ at that time. And, uh, he was, what do you say . . . helping the chauffeur. And so, well, they went to this railroad crossing and they couldn't make it in time because they said that the truck died there—just stopped. By the time they knew that the train was coming, it just hit the truck. I had my little girl already and I was pregnant at the time. That's when everything started, instead of me being happy, I started being unhappy.

DOCTOR: You were pretty happy at that time?

PATIENT: Um hm. But then, like I say, everything was . . . I don't know; it's been too mixed up (laughs).

DOCTOR: Well . . .

PATIENT: I don't really know how to explain it.

DOCTOR: Well, I imagine it's awful hard to explain, and you don't have to explain it all here to us. I guess you got pretty depressed at that time, kind of blue and upset?

PATIENT: Yeah. It's like I say, like at the time when he was killed, I didn't even know that he had an accident 'til . . . the accident happened around 12 noon and I didn't know until about 2:00 in the evening. That's when a man from the company came and told me that my husband had an accident. But he didn't tell me that he was dead or anything. When I got to the hospital I just went in there and they told me that I couldn't see him anymore because he was gone already. And then I didn't remember anything else until I found myself in a little room where everybody was giving me some air and everything.

DOCTOR: Yeah. Did that kind of change your life a little? I mean, the way you thought about things?

PATIENT: Well, I was pretty young at the time. I was about 16 then and I don't think that I took things real serious then.

(Each time the patient comes close to realizing strong feeling, particularly anger, she backs off. Sixteen-year-olds do have deep feelings, but we accept the patient's statement about how she felt when she was sixteen. She is not ready to talk about these feelings.)

DOCTOR: I see.

PATIENT: When I started feeling bad about things that happened to me was when I was about 20. That's when I started feeling when somebody was against me and when somebody was not.

DOCTOR: Um hm, um hm.

PATIENT: Everything, you know, that I felt that was worse than anything else was when . . . from my twentieth birthday until now.

DOCTOR: So you didn't worry much when you were younger, like that, huh?

PATIENT: No.

DOCTOR: Yeah. How do things look to you for the future?

PATIENT: Well, I don't have too much hopes, 'cause it's like I say, well my second child, he's 16 right now, and when he wants to go to school, he'll go. When he don't want, he don't go.

DOCTOR: So he's not going right now?

PATIENT: And, then I ask for help from people that I think could help me and they say, well, we can't do anything about it because they're over age and once they get to the age of 17, well, we can't do anything about it. Well, like it's been about three weeks that we started a quarrel, me and my son, just because of a glass of milk.

DOCTOR: Started what?

PATIENT: A quarrel. In the morning when he was about to go to school, I heard that he was going around with a bunch of guys real early because he used to leave real early in the morning and by the time he would go to school, he would have about an hour between classes and the time he left home. And I heard he was going around smoking with these kids and everything and they didn't even know what they were smoking, but they were smoking. And 'cause I don't let him smoke at home, you know, in front of me. And . . . or I told him that if he wanted to smoke, just to let me know and I would go ahead and let him smoke. So he don't do it in front of me anyway. So that time I told him that I wanted him not to go to school so early and he says, well, I want to go down there because I want to have some breakfast. I says, well, we can have breakfast here. He says, no, I'm going down to school. I says no, you're not going to school this early. You're going to eat your breakfast here. Then he started talking and yelling back at me and I told him, don't yell at me. He says, well, I need some milk to drink in the mornings and you don't have milk here. I said, there's a glass out there and that's enough for you to drink. He said no, I don't want a glass, I want two glasses. So, well . . . shut up and I started toward him and by the time I knew it we were fighting. I didn't talk to him because I told him that if he didn't ask forgiveness I wasn't going to talk to him and he wasn't going to receive nothing from me. He wouldn't do it. And he's a very stubborn boy (laugh). So, I say that now I have problems, but I don't take them that serious.

(Again, she backs away from feelings.)

DOCTOR: Try to let them wash off, huh?

PATIENT: Yeah (laughs).

DOCTOR: How about the next one down?

PATIENT: Oh, the next one, he's 14.

DOCTOR: Is he in school?

PATIENT: He's going to school. He don't miss school. He tries his best to study. Instead of me having to give him money to go to the movie, he says to save it and he goes to his classes. Or, like whenever they have a movie at school, they need money, and he says, no, I don't need money, I'm going to a class instead. He's a real good boy. And the third one, he's pretty good too. They're still studying.

DOCTOR: They're working hard?

PATIENT: Um hm. Couse they've never been out of my sight. They've always been by me and everything.

DOCTOR: Um hm.

PATIENT: Since they were born until now. But these two oldest ones . . . well, I think that was the main problem. I left them out of my sight. Because my mother took them to Chicago and she had them down there for a while and then she brought them back when she couldn't handle them anymore. She said they were too much work for her and all that.

DOCTOR: She brought them back?

(Did separation from mother and her emotional unavailability because of the death of her first husband have anything to do with the problems of the older children?)

PATIENT: Um hm.

DOCTOR: That was what you were telling me you were worried about before . . . that she might take the others too?

PATIENT: Um hm.

DOCTOR: I see.

PATIENT: Well, like right now. Everybody's at home and we're real well organized. Like I say, since those three don't leave me alone, I think I'm all right.

(There was a pause here and we need to know more about past history.)

DOCTOR: Are you from this city?

PATIENT: Yes, I was born here.

DOCTOR: And how far did you go in school?

PATIENT: To the third grade.

(This is a good example of how education does not necessarily coincide with intelligence and abstracting ability. She is an intelligent woman, even though she only completed the third grade. She grasps the abstract and complicated concept that how one feels about oneself and others relates to eating habits and relationships in the outside world.)

DOCTOR: Third grade. And then what?

PATIENT: My mother and father were having problems. One went this way and the other went that way. So, we usually went back and forth. We didn't have a steady place to stay, so one month in one school, one month in another. And by the time I knew it, we were working out in the fields and I said, well, I'd better stop going to school because . . . anyway, we don't get enough studying and everything.

DOCTOR: Did you go out from here to work in the fields?

PATIENT: No. They used to take us out there to live with our grandmother.

DOCTOR: Um hm. Well, I guess there are a lot of things we could talk about here, but is it time for us to stop?

(This was admittedly too abrupt.)

I want to ask you just one question before we stop and that is, if you could say what would be the most help to you—things are going pretty well, but you have quite a few problems, I know, and you've told us about some of them—what would be the most help to you?

PATIENT: What would make me more happier?

DOCTOR: Yeah.

PATIENT: For her to return to school.

DOCTOR: In other words, if there were some way that you could help her to be happier and get back in school, that'd be the thing that you'd want most.

PATIENT: Um hm.

DOCTOR: Okay. Well, we'll stop and let you go now. Thank you very much.

A reminder: In spite of all myths, we have no way of knowing what is in another person's mind. We can only provide the opportunity for the person to tell us.

Index